THE SIRTFOOD DIET 2020

The Revolutionary Method Used By Celebrities For Fast Weight Loss, Stay Fit And Live Healthy

By

Susan Strasmore

and utter responsibility of the recipient reader. Under no circumstances will any legal responsibility or blame be held against the publisher for any reparation, damages, or monetary loss due to the information herein, either directly or indirectly.

Respective authors own all copyrights not held by the publisher.

The information herein is offered for informational purposes solely, and is universal as so. The presentation of the information is without contract or any type of guarantee assurance.

The trademarks that are used are without any consent, and the publication of the trademark is without permission or backing by the trademark owner. All trademarks and brands within this book are for clarifying purposes only and are the owned by the owners themselves, not affiliated with this document.

AUTHOR'S EXPERIENCE ON SIRT FOOD DIET

Because I do even better because I have a schedule, I decided that I wanted one to keep on board and find something who might work for me. I figured Whole 30 wasn't going to work this weekend, but this weekend, reading an article regarding Sirtfood Diet lists the healthy options of coffee, chocolate, and red wine. (feels amazing already). Sounds nice now. Aidan, a pharmacologist, and Glen, who is an MA in nutritional medicine, met in 2012 when they published a criticism of the supplement industry – The Health Delusion – where they revealed how millions of us take vitamin pills that we don't need and in some instances they can be positively unhealthy since they provide a much higher dosage of nutrients than a And the pair recently started to study sirtuins. So, what are sirtuins exactly, and how do they motivate me to lose weight?

Sirtuins are a protein class present in living organisms engaged in metabolic processes. 'Sirtfoods' have a high level of sirtuin and replicate the effects of exercise and fasting through muscle increment, fat-burning, increasing muscle, and staving disease. They store sirtuins foods like green tea, kale, and apples to stimulate "skinny" genetic-pathways and help you lose fat as fast as possible.

The top ten Sirtfoods are the following:

Blueberries, Parsley, Capers, Citrus seeds, Coffee, Red Wine, Green Tea, dark chocolate

The plan appeared to be comfortable enough, drinking three SIRT juices three times a day for the first 3-days, then eating dinner. Also, drink 2-SIRT fluids per day in days 4-7 and eat 2 sorts of food. The report stated that almost all interested in the program dropped at least 7lbs within seven days. I've converted to juice now, so this aspect was protected, so it seemed like I might get behind a program when you are permitted coffee, red wine, so Dark Chocolate.

As the book wasn't published until today, I used the recipes in this book to continue with myself and imagine what tiny amounts is intended by this, my week is so far ... My days were all the same, wake up, drink tea, and some lemon. Have an espresso a little later, and then try waiting till 10 am until I drink my first juice, and when I eat it with a bit of quantity of protein (not on schedule), try reducing the sugar absorbance from the liquid.

Monday – Drink lots, tea, espresso, one taste SIRT juice 3 Times regular, (a mini bit of protein: 1 hard-boiled white egg, 1 3 oz chick part and one handful of cooked edamame), 85% dark chocolate and dinner Sirt – 100% veggie and potatoes (recipe next week)

I needed a snack, but not because I was starving ... only because I used to snack every day. NO hunger pains and I was full to the gills during dinner. Buckwheat pasta was first sampled, and I loved it ...... as did the hubby (he was shocked).

Tuesday – Coffee, tea, expressos, 1 cup of SIRT juice three times a day, (3 little bits of protein two hard-boiled egg whites and 1 3 oz chicken portion), a small square (10 g) of 85% of Lindt, Dark chocolate, sort food dinner – spiced couscous with capers, psalm and bowl (can go vegan or use shrimp) – baked next week, served in a healthy manner

No pains of hunger and couldn't finish juice # 3, drank only half. When dinner rolls around, the plan says that I'm hungry after 7:30 pm. The dinner was another home-course dessert (even the hubby liked it), and I ended up with a whole butt. Slept like a little kid and slept healthier than I had in months!

Wednesday – 1 L coffee, tea, 1 cup of Sirt juice two times a day, two tiny pieces of protein (1 hardboiled egg white and 3 oz chicken portion), dark chocolate cube, red wine * with 6 oz.

No hunger pains again. I was so thorough that I was unable to drink my 3rd juice every day – instead, I chose an early meal and bed at 9:30 am instead of the usual 11:00 pm (since I had an early morning today). I made my sort of food meal for dinner, and it was delicious again. I continue to think this mission has been made for me ...

I wanted to get on the scale the next morning, which is on *Thursday*. I knew I felt good, and I slept better, and I got less bloated, and so I was hopeful but not too excited ... I was 2.75 pounds in three days, but it was even more astonishing to get more than a half-pound of muscle! Again, I weighed to be satisfied, and it was right. I write this book on my face with a big grin and feel fantastic.

One outcome of this program is my excellent blood sugar control – I haven't got lower or dense and have the best numbers in months at present!

TABLE OF CONTENTS

INTRODUCTION

Adele's weight loss has all the people can think and talk about lately, particularly after pictures of the singer appear on the Oscars after-party, reportedly seven-stone lighter.

This comes after photos of the singer who has lost three stones on a beach in Anguilla at Christmas.

When Adele debuted her slimmer appearance at the Billboard Music Awards in May, the Sirtfood diet started to get known. Her chef and trainer, Pete Geracimo, is a big culinary fan and claims the singer lost 30 pounds to Sirtfood.

How did she do it? It seems that by taking up the Sirtfood Diet – famous for actively promoting red wine and chocolate for those who adopt it.

In recent years, the Sirtfood diet is widely known, and it is as popular as the Cabbage Soup diet of Adele, Dukan diet and 5.2 Diet, and famous people like Jodie Kidd and Lorraine Pascale are also common. But is it yet another diet that claims to you too much, or could it help you get lean and feel better adopting a diet plan?

SirtFood is a group of foods (relatively recently found), necessary for triggering the 'Sirtuin' genes in our bodies; these are the genes that are triggered in fasting diets. The book lists the top Sirtfoods, including bird's-eye calm, chocolate, capers, celery, cocoa, green tea, and kale, and details a 7-day diet plan that is very strong on the top 20 Sirtfoods.

This book will help you to burn fat and boost your energy and will prepare your body for long-term loss of weight and a longer, sicker, healthy life. When drinking red wine, all this. Sounds like the dream meal, right? Well, before your savings are fried with sirtuins, read and enjoy this excellent piece.

CHAPTER 1
WHAT IS SIRTFOOD?

Sirtfood diet is based on the idea that some particular foods activate sirtuins in the body, specific proteins hypothesized to reap different benefits from protecting your body's cells from inflammation to reverse aging. The diet is accompanied by items such as green tea, dark chocolate, bananas, citrus fruits, parsley, turmeric, spinach, blueberries, capers, and red wine.

Sirtfood diets proponents identify that this diet has two "simple" levels. The first phase is the seven days each day with 3-Sirtfood green juices and 1-Sirtfood meal – a total of 1000-calories. But do not discourage: you can feel much less hungry in 4th to the 7th day if you can raise your calorie consumption to 1,500-calories with 2-green juices and two meals.

Phase two is less optimistic. This is a two-week duration in which three "healthy" Sirt-food-rich meals are allowed each day, in addition to one unique green juice.

The aim is to promote more weight loss during this period. The effects of Sirtuins are exciting, but the Sirtfood diet is another way to "lose seven pounds in seven days! "And now you learn why extreme diets don't work like that.

There are three reasons for moving on the diet for Sirtfood:

1. The Sirtfood diet only measures weight loss success

The weight is a health determinant, but it is not the only one. To measure someone's fitness performance by dropping X pounds in X time, all other effects of diet are overlooked. Food is full of energy so that you can do things such as showering, exercise, and breathing. It often has nutrients that can facilitate many body functions and is also a typically enjoyable activity. There is so more much to reflect on mental wellbeing than size, and it is not sufficient to assess performance just in terms of weight loss.

2. It is restrictive that can affect your food relationship

This diet stresses a moderate intake of 1,000 to 1,500 calories, far smaller than most people require. If we severely limit the consumption of our food, our instinctive reaction is excessive. Your body is intelligent and finds this absence of food to be an assault. We appear to overcompensate, so we can all respond to "hanging" and, therefore, when we have the chance to eat. Careful and intuitive feeding is a more natural approach than reducing calories.

3. The diet for Sirtfood is not medical or science-based

While the effects of sirtuins are uncertain, the unique Sirtfood diet has little to no study. We already have those standards that have been thoroughly studied and checked for decades. This is a better place to start if you're confused about what 'healthy food' is.

It's okay in case you want to include a few Sirt menus in a food plan. Foods such as green tea, berries, dark chocolate, and cabbage have, after all, a place to eat! However, following a program with such stringent passing or failure requirements is unrealistic and could harm your food relationship. By implementing a food plan full of variation and feeding wisely, you can have a long-term, sustainable relationship with food.

Science Behind Sirtfood Diet

Since way back, people have been fascinated by the mythical fountain of young people. Rapid to the 21st century and little changed, despite a significant research curiosity centered on the family of genes that control metabolism called sirtuin and their influential behavior, which can radically alter the roles of our cells. These dominant genes help us to burn the fat, fit, and stop disease and ultimately the closest we can ever turn the clock back.

But if we find them to be 'skinny genes' or 'peter pan genes' as the media loves to spin, the unique aspect of the sirtuin is their ability to transform our cells into a survival mode. They do this by initiating a steady cycle of recycling called autophagy, which eliminates cell waste and debris that forms over time and is believed to cause 'inflammatory.' The results of this cycle of rejuvenation are impressive: our cells revert to a more youthful condition, where inflammation is decreased, fat burns rise, and we look like we do in the first period again.

What is the question of the million dollars: ways we can activate Sirtuins, then how can it make a significant difference? The two methods of exercise and fasting are well known. However, as someone would say, they can be both terrible and sometimes incompatible with our challenging 21st-century lifestyle. They are also well known for their downfalls. As many people would be aware, the reduction in Calories will make us exhausted, 'hangry.' In the longer term, the muscles will erode and allow metabolism to stagnate. The mixture is incredibly stressful and hungry. The sum required for the weight loss is Hercules, as far as exercise is concerned.

But what if there were a different, less strenuous way, a way that nature always wanted us to do?

In 2013, we reported the findings of one of the most significant game changes in our understanding of food. The most essential, best-conducted nutrition study conducted in the modern age was called PREDIMED, and it was carried out on nearly 7,500 people, posed a straightforward question: how did a special virgin Mediterranean-style diet or nuts compare to a more traditionalized western diet of walnuts or extra virgin olive oil? The result was excellent. After five years, an unprecedented 30% of diabetes and heart disease have been reduced, along with significant inflammation and obesity reduction. But it was still to come what was most impressive about this research. Upon further investigation, it was apparent that the number of calories, fat, or carbohydrates they consumed was not substantially different between the two classes. This is the standard way to determine how proper a diet is. Something different was happening, something that modern nutrition still needs to consider.

Plant nutrients, such as walnuts and virgin olive oil, contain natural compounds called polyphenols, the health advantages of which are now demonstrated through studies. The findings were surprising when researchers analyzed PREDIMED polyphenol use. Three and seven percent fewer deaths of people who consume the highest polyphenols than those who consume the least over only five years.

But not everybody is equivalent to polyphenols. For example, research carried out whereby almost 3,000 twins showed that only some polyphenols were higher intake and that the body fats were reduced and that fat was better distributed. Certain polyphenols are a boon for slender and healthier stay, but what are the best polyphenols? Will those who have demonstrated work be capable of switching on our sirtuin genes? Is it the same as fasting and exercise activated?

This concept was quickly taken up by the pharmaceutical industry, spending considerable sums to turn sirtuin-activating nutrients into panacea medicines. When Glaxo Smith Kline paid almost one billion dollars for the reserve nutrient research rights to produce a sirtuin-activating drug, it gave great impetus. They were, however, the target of isolation and pharmaceutical doses of a single nutrient, as research indicates that the benefits derived from a balance of nutrients ingested at doses that can be obtained from dietary sources.

Many people would have learned of metformin, the most common diabetes medication, and others will read it either or know anyone. It is not likely that it originates from a natural herb of French lilac and uses to treat diabetes as far ago as the 1800s. Metformin is also known as the first FDA approved drug to be investigated for life prolongation while most popular medicinal products have significant adverse effects limiting their use. And what causes that enormous advantage? We know now that metformin does not correctly function on macronutrients or blood sugar; instead, it works by stimulating the pathway of the sirtuin gene.

Paradoxically, while all over the pharmaceuticals industry, it is almost entirely unknown in the food industry to work at the genetic level to revolutionize health.

Sirtfood Diet researchers have found which foodstuffs contain the highest amount of different polyphenols shown to cause sirtuin genes in the drug tests. This resulted in defining the essential 20 Sirtfoods we put in a particular diet attentively. Extra virgin olive oil and walnuts included, just like red onions, bananas, red wine, chocolate, chilies, turmeric, green tea, and coffee. When this diet was tested, the results were incredible. On average, 7lbs in 7 days were lost to participants while their muscle mass was preserved or even increased. The best of all registered an excellent feeling, full of energy, better sleep, and significant skin changes.

Although this was a good start, the long-term results showed that these plant foods were healthy as people lost

20 to 50 pounds over 12 weeks. This included several independent studies, including a skeptic doctor recently examined on national television with his patient losing just over four weeks of a breathtaking 22 pounds. Yet weight loss is only a failure for our doctors and the wonderful foods, which work to prevent inflammation and aging at the most in-depth genetic degree in our cells. The convener of this diet found something truly unique with the change of healthy life, including people who had reversed diabetes, cardiovascular conditions, and autoimmune disorders and had the chance to leave the medication. To date, this diet (Sirtfood) has had substantial effects on a large number of people around the world, and testimonies keep coming in.

The advantages of the diet based on those foods undoubtedly show that calorie counting, carbohydrate, or banishing fat does not decide health. Nature never meant that we were healthy, based on what we cut. Instead, a character is intended to benefit us through the unparalleled pharmacy of a long and healthy life.

How Does the Sirtfood Diet Work?

The diet is divided into two stages. Stage 1: The seven-day' hyper success stage,' combines a rich Sirtfood diet with moderate calorie limitations, and step 2, which consolidates your losing weight with no calories, is the 14-day' maintenance phase.'

Phase 1

The intake of calories during the first to third day is limited to 1,000 calories (more than 5:2 fasting days). The diet is made from 3 juices high in syrup and 1 Sirt and two squares of dark chocolates. The menu is rich in green juices.

The remaining three days have increased calorie consumption to 1,500 calories, and the diet contains two green juices of Sirtfood and 2 Sirt-food-rich meals every day.

You cannot drink alcohol during phase 1, yet you can take tea, free water, coffee, and green tea.

Phase 2

Phase 2 is not about restricting calories. There are three meals rich in Sirtfood and one green juice each day and, where necessary, take one or two Sirtfood menus.

During step 2, red wine can be consumed, but with

caution (2-3 cups of red wine weekly is recommended), along with beer, tea, coffee, and green tea.

After the second phase, what happens? What about the sustainability of this type of diet?

For those who have completed the first and second stage of food, but still want to follow Sirtfood road, the idea is "Certifying." This includes taking and Sirtfood, twisting your favorite dish. Recipes include regular classics, including chicken curry, sweet chili, pizza, and pancakes.

Sirtfood Diet is not in any way a "single diet" but a way of living. You are therefore encouraged to keep consuming a rich diet of Sirtfood and drink your everyday green juice when you have successfully carried out the menu for the first three weeks. However, there are now several Sirtfood Diet recipes available with recipes for many more Sirtfood recipes; also, there are lots of methods for green juice alternatives and more tips for this diet. Sirtfood desserts even have some recipes! Phases 1 and 2, if required for an improvement in wellbeing, can be replicated if something has vanished.

Is There Any Eating Regime for Sirtfood Diet?

Sure, there is a handy map that shows you every day what you should consume. The book includes everything you need to have a successful diet plan for the first 3-weeks. A meat/fish choice is accessible every day, and a vegan/vegan alternative. Almost every meal is gluten-free, and every day there are no animal product choices so that most people have a diet.

What Will Happen After the Diet is Completed?

Sirtfood Diet is not a 'diet' but instead a way of life. This is a way of life. After you have carried out the diet plan for the first three weeks, you are advised to start consuming a diet high in Sirtfoods and keep drinking your green juice daily. The book contains recipes for some Sirtfood-rich food, recipes for some alternatives to green extract, and more essential tips and recommendations for the Sirtfood diet plan. Sirtfood desserts do have several tips! The first and second phases can be replicated if required to enhance your health or get a little out of line.

So, Will the Diet Work for Sirtfood?

Ok, according to their other widespread approvals, they've all been supported by this diet. But my favorite endorsement is probably the one I can categorically talk about.

However, I'm a bit skeptical – perhaps the food works for a celebrity who is personally coached on a diet and certainly also a personalized trainer. But will an ordinary person like me execute the Sirtfood diet plan? Ok, the query can only be addressed one way. I agreed to observe steps 1 and 2 of the Sirtfood Diet for the next three weeks and discuss how it will go.

Is Diet Effective?

The Sirtfood Diet writers say confidently that the plan will overwhelm weight loss, turn on the "skinny gene" or avoid diseases.

There is no data to help them. The question is.

There is no compelling proof to date that Sirtfood Diet does better than any other calorie-limited diet to support weight loss.

And while all of these products have medicinal properties, no long-term clinical trials have been done to establish if a diet that is high in Sirt products has any tangs.

The participants observed the diet for one week and performed it every day. At the weekend, the total loss was 7lbs (3.2 kg), and lean muscle mass was preserved or even gained.

However, these are not unexpected tests. Limitation of the calorie intake to 1,000 calories and joint exercise almost always leads to a loss of weight.

When the body is drained of nutrition, in addition to consuming fat and tissue, it uses the emergency energy reserves of glycogen.

Every glycogen molecule requires the storage of 3-4 water molecules. This even gets rid of this acid as the body utilizes glycogen. It's called the "weight of the bath."

Just about one-third of the weight reduction comes from fat in the first week of severe calorie restriction, while the other 2/3 from the skin, muscle, and glycogen.

As your calorie consumption increases, your body replenishes its glycogen stores, and the weight returns immediately.

Unfortunately, this sort of calorie restriction can decrease the body's metabolic rate, which ensures that you require fewer calories a day than ever before for energy.

Hopefully, this lifestyle will shed a few pounds at first, which will also increase as soon as the lifestyle comes to an end.

Three weeks probably aren't long enough for disease prevention to have a measurable long-term effect.

On the other side, Sirtfood may be a smart thing to introduce to the daily diet in the long run. However, you might still miss your meal, and now you will continue to do so.

Summarily, this diet will help you lose weight, but the pressure will regain when the menu ends. The list is too brief to affect your wellbeing for an extended period.

CHAPTER 2

HOW TO FOLLOW SIRTFOOD DIET

The two stages of this diet in the last three weeks in all. You should then proceed to "serve" the eating of as many Sirtfoods menus as possible in milk.

Detailed recipes for all these processes can be found in the book Sirtfood Diet, which the makers of the diet have written. To follow your diet, you must purchase it.

The meal plans are full of the diet recipes but include just the top 20-Sirtfoods, as well as other ingredients.

It is easy to find most ingredients and Sirt milk.

For these two processes, three of the required signature ingredients – Matcha green tea powder, lovage, and buckwheat – may be costly or hard to locate.

The green juice that you would produce between 1-3 times per day is a large part of the diet. The juicer and the cuisine are required as the products are indicated by weight (a blender does not work). The following is the recipe:

Sirtfood Green Juice

- 75g (2.5 oz) of kale powder

- 30g of arugula (rocket)

- 5g of parsley

- 2 pieces of celery

- 1cm of ginger

- Medium green apple

- Medium lemon

- Half tsp of Matcha green tea

Juice and pour into a glass all ingredients, except green tea powder and lemon. Pour all the lemon juice and the green tea paste from the liquid by hand. Shake the lemon by hand.

First Step

The first stage takes seven days and involves a limited amount of calorie and green juice. This aims to start your weight loss and predict that you will drop 7 lbs (3,2 kg).

The calorie intake is limited to 1000 calories in the first three days of the first phase: four green drinks a day and one meal you have to consume. Every day you can choose the recipes in the book, all of which include Sirt stuff.

The Sirt-omelet, miso-glazed tofu, or a lunch of buckwheat noodles are examples of meals.

Calorie intake is raised to 1,500 in days 4–7 of step one. You can choose two green juices per day and another two Sirt items from the journal.

Second Step

The second phase lasts two weeks. You should continue to lose weight steadily during this "maintenance" stage.

For this step, there is no clear calorie cap. Alternatively, three Sirt foods are consumed each day, and green juice is eaten each day. The food is again picked from the book's recipes.

After the Sirtfood Diet

You can replicate these two steps for more weight reduction as much as you like.

However, after these phases, you are advised to "supporting" your diet with daily Sirt menus.

There are several books on the Sirtfood Diet full of sort food recipes. Sirtfood may also be in our everyday diet as a snack.

Therefore, regular use of green juice is promoted.

The Sirtfood Diet thus is more of a transformation inhabits than a specific meal.

Summarily, the two stages of this diet. Phase 1 lasts seven days, mixing calorie restriction with natural juices. The second stage lasts two weeks and contains three meals and one sauce.

What To Eat on Sirtfood Diet

The headlines in Sirtfood Diet are red wine and dark chocolate because they are high in Sirtuin's activator.

While this is not the entire picture, so by the line Merlot so Green & Blacks (more pity), you do not notice the impact.

The Sirtfood Diet program intends to increase consumption. Those are as follows:

- Apple

- Citrus fruits

- Red wine

- Walnuts

- Buckwheat

- Medjool dates

- Dark chocolate

- Capers

- Parsley

- Soy

- Green tea

- Blueberries

- Olive oil

- Turmeric

- Strawberries

- Kale

- Red onion

- Rocket

Curiously, coffee is another fantastic sort of food that is excellent news if you're scared to have caffeine cut out. Both Japan and Italy are consistently listed among the world's healthiest countries, where people consume a large number of Sirt foods already.

Is Sirtfoods the Latest Superfoods?

Nobody should doubt that sirtfood is perfect for you. The nutrients and safe compounds are often substantial.

However, several of the items on the Sirtfood Diet indicated were related to health benefits in research.

For example, a moderately high cocoa content in dark chocolate will lessen the risk of having heart ailment and help fight inflammation.

Green tea can also help in lowering blood pressure, minimize the risk of stroke and diabetes.

So, turmeric has anti-inflammatory features that favor the body broadly and may also guard against chronic inflammatory diseases.

Currently, certain sirtfoods have demonstrated safety benefits for humans.

There is, however, insufficient proof of the safety effects of elevated amounts of a sirtuin protein. However, animal and cell lines research has produced exciting findings.

Scientists also discovered, for instance, that elevated rates of some sirtuin proteins enable the yeast, mice, and mouse to live longer.

Sirtuin proteins often teach the body to eat more fat for energy and increase insulin responsiveness through fasting or calorie restriction. One mice research found that higher levels of Sirtuin contributed to fat loss.

Other research suggests that sirtuins can also help minimize inflammation, prevent tumor growth, and delay cardiac disease and Alzheimer's progress.

While studies have demonstrated positive results in mice and human cell lines, no social studies have demonstrated the effects of increasing levels of Sirtuin.

It is unclear whether growing amounts of Sirtuin-protein in our body contribute to a longer life or less cancer risk in humans.

Work on creating compounds successful at rising amounts of Sirtuin in the body is currently underway. Human studies can thus begin to explore the health effects of sirtuins.

Before then, the consequences of elevated sirtuin rates cannot be calculated.

However, sort food is usually healthy. Nevertheless, there is little or no information as to how sirtuin rates and human health impact these products.

Are Sirtfoods Healthy and Sustainable?

Nearly all are safe, and even its antioxidant or anti-inflammatory properties will contribute to certain health benefits.

Yet eating only a few particularly healthy foods cannot meet every nutritional requirement of your body.

The diet is unnecessary and does not offer any clear and unique health benefits compared with any other type of food.

Besides, it is typically not recommended to eat only

1,000 calories without physician supervision. Many people are overly restrictive in consuming 1,500 calories per day.

Also, up to 3 green juices, a day is required for the diet. While these juices can be a great source of minerals and vitamins, they do contain virtually no healthy fiber from whole fruits and vegetables. They are a source of sugar too.

Moreover, sipping tea all day long is a terrible thing for blood sugar and teeth alike.

It is also more than likely a lack of proteins, vitamins, and minerals, especially during the first stage, since the diet is so limited in food choice and calories.

This diet may be hard to stick to for three weeks because of the limited food choices and low calories.

Connect it to the very initial costs of buying a juicer, the book, and some unusual, pricey products and time to prepare specific foods and juices, and many people find the lifestyle to be unfeasible and impractical.

However, the diet promotes balanced but reduces food choices and calories. There is also a lot of juice to drink, which is not a strong recommendation.

Safety and Side Effects

With a low or incomplete nutritional content and low calories, the first phase of the Sirtfood Diet does not present any safety measures for an average, healthy adult as the diet takes shorter periods.

However, a person with diabetes may cause dangerous changes in blood sugar levels, with a reduction in calories, mainly with a savor's drinking.

However, some side effects can even occur to a healthy person — mostly hunger.

Eating just 1,000–1,500 calories a day can leave virtually everyone starving, especially if you are consuming juice that is low in fiber, a nutrient that allows you to feel complete.

Many side-effects, such as exhaustion, lighting, and irritability, may arise during Step One because of the calorie restriction.

When the lifestyle is practiced only for three weeks, the customarily balanced person may have serious health implications.

The diet is inadequate in calories, and the first step is not nutritionally equilibrated. It might leave you hungry, but for a typical stable person, it's not risky.
28

CHAPTER 3
SIRTFOODS DIET HEALTH BENEFITS

Sirtuin activators are gradually seen to have a wide variety of health effects, including muscle strengthening hunger suppression. It enhances the body's function, boosts blood sugar levels, and removes the harm done by free radical molecules that can build up in cells and contribute to cancer and other diseases.

Professor Frank Hu, a professional in nutrition and epidemiology at Harvard University, said in a recent article in the journal Advances In nutrition, 'There is a piece of significant evidence for the beneficial effect of intake of food and drink that is rich in sirtuin activators, reducing the risk from chronic illness' An anti-aging diet for Sirtfoods is particularly suitable.

While Sirtuin activators exist throughout the entire herb realm, there is ample Sirtfood for some fruits and vegetables. Examples include green tea, cocoa powder, turmeric, almonds, onions, and pork.

Most of the items on sale, including strawberries, avocados, bananas, lettuce, kiwis, carrots, and cucumber, in supermarkets are also very low in the amount of Sirtuins on show. That does not say that they are not worth eating since they give several other benefits.

It's a lot more versatile than other diets as it consumes a diet filled with Sirtfood. You should only consume a few Sirtfoods healthily. Or in a focused form, you might get them. The 5:2 menu could require extra calories on low-calorie days if you incorporate Sirt products.

One surprising conclusion from one Sirtfood diet trial is that participants lose significant muscle weight. In reality, participants were often muscled, which contributed to a more refined and toned appearance. This is the uniqueness of Sirtfoods; fat burning is enabled, thus sustaining, maintaining, and repairing muscles. It compares completely with other diets where the loss of fat and muscle usually occurs, with muscle loss slowing down metabolism and rendering weight gain more possible.

There are seven Sirtuins, numbered SIRT1 through SIRT7, and while all seven have not been shown to be effective, evidence suggests that their activation can aid in the following ways.

- **Helps Control Weight**

Lab-based experiments have not only demonstrated how treatments with trigger Sirtuins contribute to substantially lower body weights, but also that even amid a high-fat diet, Sirtuins successfully shield against weight gain.

- **Improves Memory**

Besides defending neurons from disorders like Alzheimer 's, the Sirtuins often enhance memory and learning by improving synaptic plasticity or how well the brain's neurons may adapt their links to new information. In addition to protecting neurons from injury.

- **Protect Against Diabetes**

An elevated sirtuin development, lowers a significant risk ofType 2 diabetes, has shown a safety against insulin resistance. Likewise, reduced sirtuin production brings about an increased risk of diabetes. Cells become more sensitive to insulin so that more glucose from the bloodstream can be eliminated. If you note that the key to diabetes and weight gain is insulin resistance, it may be good news for your butt.

- **Helps Fight Cancer**

Chemicals that act as activators inhibit the way sirtuins work in different cells and activate them in healthy and normal cells, yet disconnect them from cancer cells that encourage them to die.

- **Slow down the Ageing Process**

Several animal-based studies link sirtuin-activating proteins with a healthier, longerexistence. Researchers say it is because Sirtuins protect cells and slower the age of cells as guardian enzymes.

However, a lot of other health benefits also come into play with SIRTUINS.

- **Sleep**

The activation of Sirtuins helps you to create sleep and wake hormones at your circadian rhythm.

- **Memory**

The turmeric from Sirtfood has demonstrated short-term memory improvement and protection from cognition problems. Put this in for a brainier start to the day with your morning coffee.

Sirtuins Enhances Your Body's Wellness Genes

The "Fountain of Youth" and how we would lead happier and safer lives have also intrigued us. Ok, a gene family called the Sirtuins has the same interest in the scientific community. We each contain Sirtuins – often called our skinny genes – and they are really fascinating. They have the power to determine matters such as our ability to stay slim and burn fat, our sensitivity to diseases, and even how long we can live.

So how strong are Sirtuins? Because they can turn our cells into a type of survival mode, Sirtuins are particularly capable of leading to a potent recycling process that clears cell waste and fats. The advantages are quite spectacular: fat melts away, and we are fitter, leaner, and healthier.

How Do We Profit from Sirtuins?

What can we do to enhance Sirtuins and reap these incredible benefits? Fasting and exercise are well known to trigger the Sirtuins. Unfortunately, they also claim a firm commitment to food restrictions or rigorous exercise regimes. Reduced calorie rates make us feel tired, hungry, and profoundly cranky and can induce muscle loss and slow metabolism in the longer term. For example, it requires a lot energy and dedication to ensure that the amount required for weight loss is successful. Both can be difficult to achieve.

Not Every (Healthy) Food is Produced in Equal Measure

Study now shows that plants contain natural compounds known as polyphenols, which have huge health benefits. And the results were stunning when researchers who analyzed PREDIMED studied the consumption of polyphenol among the participants. Those who ingest the highest polyphenol levels was 30% fewer deaths over the five years compared with those who ingest the least.

However, not all polyphenol is the same. Harvard University studies from more than 124,000 individuals have shown that weight management can only be achieved by certain polyphenols. Similarly, a survey of close to 3,000 twins has shown that only some polyphenols have a higher intake with a healthier fat distribution. Surely polyphenols are an excellent way to stay healthy and slim, but in case they aren't all fair, who is the best? Could those who have been investigated be able to switch on our sirtuin genes? The same ones that are triggered by fasting and training?

Such sirtuin-activating compounds have already been used by the pharmaceutical sector to spend hundreds of millions to make them panacea. The most famous diabetes medication metformin, for example, originates from a plant that stimulates our sirtuin genes. Until now, the field of eating, to the disadvantage of our well-being and our waistlines, has largely disregarded them.

What Foods Activate Sirtuins?

We also placed all the foodstuffs with the largest sirtuin triggering polyphenols in a particular diet together with our curiosity. It contains olive oil and walnuts, red onions, tomatoes, red wines, dark chocolate, green tea, and several more items. The results were amazing when we pilot-tested it. Participants lost weight while maintaining their muscle mass or even increasing it. Best of all, people reported that they looked great — with stamina, more sleep, and significant skin changes.

So was introduced the Sirtfood Diet, a groundbreaking new way for Sirtuins to be stimulated by tasty food. A diet without calorie counting, carbohydrate, or low-fat intake. A balanced lifestyle in which you take advantage of consuming your love food. The Sirtfood Diet challenges the condition of healthy food counseling and what it means to feel good and look good. Everything from our favorite foods

Losing Weight with Sirtfood Diet

The triggering of the SIRT genes triggers a metabolic shift that breaks down more fat cells. The enabled SIRTs to increase the amount of norepinephrine named neurotransmitters used by the nervous system to trigger fat cells to break down fat. The signal that the fat cell transforms fat into energy becomes greater and fat consumes more and more. This is the way to help you with Sirtfoods lose weight. The weight-loss studies in foods that contain fat is at the fore-front of new study in this area to lose weight with this diet.

Would you like to burn more fat?

Get some green tea. SIRT activators paired with a (small) dose of caffeine are mixed with green tea. The role of the SIRTs is improved by caffeine, which eliminates more fat.

When our body breakdown fat and fat is transformed into electricity, a common suppressive appetite effect exists. The body immediately uses this electricity. This has a good impact on the way you act, raising your levels of energy and rising hunger feelings.

Turning weight into muscle

The combination of SIRTs and preparation further improves the fat-burning benefit. If you exercise fat cell capacity, the power of your muscles is usable.

In practice, this means you not only lower your weight but also look leaner because some flesh has been converted into muscle when following this diet and exercising several times a week.

Drink 2-3 cups of green tea (for SIRTs and caffeine) within an hour before or after exercise to reach total optimum fat-burning efficiency.

Sirtfoods or Supplements

In the field of nutrition science, Sirtuin activators and Sirtfood are very new. A 'Sirtfood' is a nutrient-rich in the activators of Sirtuins. Vitamins, vitamins 50 years ago and Sirtuin activators just over ten years ago were found over 100 years ago.

Resveratrol, found on red grape skin (that is why red wine is supposed to keep you healthy), pomegranates, and Japanese weeds were the first activator to be identified, and still the best-known activator.

There came quickly other Sirtuin activators such as catechin (found in green tea to interact with cancer cells) and cacao powder epicatechin (responsible for the nutritional benefits of dark chocolate).

However, work has already begun after GlaxoSmithKline, the pharmaceutical company, acquired the generic resveratrol form rights. It was pleased that the findings were not spectacular but a cancer procedure. The company announced in 2010 that the research had stopped.

But now it seems that consuming this diet that is essentially rich in Sirtuin activators may be an alternative to safer, more efficient, and cheaper drugs. That was why the Sirtfood and diet had been several recent trials. Current findings show that Sirtfoods go precisely in the same direction as calorie restriction and exercise to reduce weight and stay safe.

Sirtfoods and Other Diets?

Not only is Sirtfood endorsed by all other nutritional practices, but it also significantly increases their wellbeing and weight effects. This applies to diets that are currently extremely popular like paleo, intermittent fasting, low carbon, and gluten-free.

The ingestion of a diet rich in Sirtfoods-diet would result in a decrease in calorie limits on intermittent fasting but will have same if not more significant benefits. A gain of 7 days rather than just 5 on the fasting scheme of 5:2 days.

Sirtfood can dramatically increase low-carb diets without plant-based foods. A lot of the top-20 Sirtfood products are low in carbohydrates.

Sirtfoods are paleo-typical foods that contain the polyphenols which trigger the sirtuin that people have eaten and reaped the benefits of many years. Sirtfood is a paleo ideology lacking.

The top 20-Sirtfoods are gluten-free, which makes them useful to all people who adopt a gluten-free diet.

Vegetarians & Vegans

Whereas vegans and vegetarians can benefit from all the advantages of a Sirtfood diet, attention must be paid to nutrients that are not available, and appropriate food choices or even supplements may be needed. There is a chance of dietary deficiency without animal protein to support Sirtfoods.

These are the places for those who use a herbal diet and seek additional support from the Sirtfood menu.

- Fatty acids

- Omega-3 fatty acids

- Vitamin B12

- Iodine

- Calcium

The study on the possible deficiencies of food choices is generally well known among vegetarian and dairy.

CHAPTER 4
LOSING 7 POUNDS IN 7-DAYS MEAL PLAN

Without giving up chocolate and wine Sirtfood Diet can help you lose 7-lbs in 7 days.

A Bit of Science: Why Sirtfoods are Special

Sirtfoods have recently been discovered as an activator group of plants that switch on our 'skinny' genes, the same genes activated by training and fasting, called Sirtuin Activators.

In addition to the fat-burning effect, sirtfoods are also unique in their ability to regulate their appetite naturally and increase their muscles, making them the perfect solution for healthy weight.

Their effects on health are so strong that studies have demonstrated their efficacy in preventing chronic conditions, which is more effective than prescription drugs, with visible effects on diabetes, heart disease, and the disease of his family.

Not surprisingly, Sirtfoods from cultures – such as Japan and Italy – are the world's cleanest and healthiest. So, we have built a lifestyle for them for this purpose.

Sirtfood List

Both Sirtfoods are readily available, and all products are readily available. These include red wine, dark chocolate, black coffee, Kale, rocket, coffee, petty ointments, fresh wines, olive oil extra virgin walnuts, spices, celcry, chili, apples, and buckwheat: blueberries, black tea, celeries.

What is the proof?

Our diets were explicitly evaluated for research and improving health in a gym in South West London. The tests were fantastic for us. Typically, in seven days, participants lost 7lbs, and muscle mass, well-being, and energy increased.

However, I expected people to lose some weight but never expected it to be so much, nor to retain and even gain muscle, which is very rare in the diet.

Top Sirtfoods

Some of the most substantial things you want to incorporate to your diet are:

- Buckwheat

- Capers

- Celery

- Chili

- Chocolate

- Extra Virgin Olive Oil

- Coffee

- Green Tea – ideally Matcha

- Kale

- Lovage

- Medjool Dates

- Parsley

- Red Chicory

- Red Onion

- Red Wine

- Rocket

- Soy

- Strawberries

- Turmeric

- Walnuts

Getting Started

Juicer to make the needed daily green juices is the single kit you need to keep with Sirtfood diets. While we're dreaming about the right juicers, we aren't stuck on that too much. You can only manage to get one.

You may also need to purchase some green Matcha tea powder to attach fat-burning Sirtfoods to your juices. One remedy is to hold the dust out of the water, but not as strong, and to drink 2-3 cups of green tea every day.

MEAL PLANNER

Sirtfood diet is based on a three-week two-stage scheme. The first week is a seven-day intensive program aiming at starting weight loss.

Weeks 2&3 are a continuing weight-loss maintenance program (1-2 lbs a week expected) and health changes.

Below is a meal plan, select which you will like to go for:

WEEK 1:

Day 1 – 3: (1,000 calories/day)

- ***Breakfast:*** Green juice

- ***Mid-**morning: Green juice

- ***Dinner:***15-20g of chocolate

Day 4 – 3: (1,500 calorie/day)

Prepare as described; however, you remove one of the three green juices for a second-day meal – below for breakfast or lunch.

WEEK 2 & 3 (No calorie counted):

Each day should the following:

- 3 x primary Sirtfood meals

- 1 green juice Sirtfood

- 2 snacks, pick a couple of the walnuts, strawberries or blueberries or an apple

Breakfasts:

- Green juice (see the following recipe)

- Omelet Sirtfood – ham, chicory, parsley.

- Greek yogurt-chop 10 g dark grated chocolate, walnuts chopped and mixed berries

- Spiced chilly and turmeric scrambled eggs

Lunches:

- Fried black fried cabbage

- Chili with baked potato vegetables and kidney beans

- Green onion, celery, apples, and pasta Waldorf meal.

- Walnut, pesto and red onion salad baked chicken breast

Dinners:

- Buckwheat noodles ground stir-fry (see recipe below) •

- Basil and chili-salsa chicken breast

- Fillet of chicory salmon, rocket and salad of celery

- Red wine beef, rings of onions, roasted herb potatoes.

- Bean stew from Tuscany

SIRT FOOD GREEN JUICE

Purification: Sirtfood Green Juice

- Two large handfuls or 75g of Kale

- A large handful or 30g of rocket

- A tiny handful or 5g flat-leaf Parsley

- 2–3 big stalk or 150g (including the leaves)

- Half a green apple

- Juice of half lemon with a half teaspoon of Matcha

Instruction:

1. Juice all but the green tea ingredients. Mix a little liquid in a bottle and put a fork and pour the remainder of the juice into the drink again. Then blend the Matcha.

2. In a single batch of morning, you will make up all your natural juices and relax until you need it.

PRAWN STIR FRY WITH NOODLES

Healthy: Prawn Stir-fry with Noodles

- 150g shelled raw prawns

- 2 tablespoons of soy sauce

- 2 tsp of olive oil extra virgin.

- 75g of soba

- 1 pickled clove of garlic

- 1 bird-eye chili

- 1 tsp of fresh ginger finely cut

- Sliced 20g red onions

- Sliced, 40g of celery

- 75g of green bean (sliced)

- 50g of Kale (chopped)

- 100ml chicken stock

Instruction:

1. Cook the creams with 1 tsp of soy and 1 tsp of oil and put them on a hand for 2 minutes. Cook the noodles on the packet as instructed. Drain and store.

2. Then, fry the remainder of the oil and veggie spices for 2–3 minutes over medium-high heat. Put the stock and then let it simmers till the veggies are crunchy but still tender, and then cool for 1 or 2 minutes.

3. Attach to the bowl the prawns and noodles, return to the simmer. Take it away from the source of heat and then serve.

BEEF WITH ONION RINGS, HERB ROASTED POTATOES, AND RED WINE

Hearty: Beef with Onion Rings, Herb Roasted Potatoes and Red Wine

- 100g of potatoes-peeled and diced
- 1 tbsp of olive oil extra virgin
- 5g of finely chopped Parsley

- 50g of sliced rings red onions

- 50g of chopped Kale

- One clove of garlic-thinly hacked

- 100g beef steak

- 40ml of red wine

- One tablespoon of tomato puree

- 100ml of beef stock

- One tablespoon of cornflour dissolved in water

Instruction:

1. To 220C / gas 7, heat the ovens. Boil the potatoes, then rinse, for 5 minutes. Set in 1-tsp of oil and fry for 35-45 minutes. Turn every 10 minutes and turn every 10 minutes. Take off the chopped Parsley, then blend well when baked.

2. Fry onion for 5–7 minutes in 1 tablespoon of oil, until well caramelized, and then medium heat. Drain the Kale and steam for 2-3 minutes. In ½-tsp of oil, gently cook garlic for 1-minute,

till you notice the smoothness, attach the chicken and fry until tender, for another 1-2 minutes.

3. Cook beef over medium heat with 1⁄2 teaspoon oil and fried in a hot pot, as you like frying it. Take it out of the saucepan and set aside.

4. In the warm bowl, halve the wine into the pan until squashy. Then, you can add stock and tomato-purée and then boil and thicken a little by the time the cornflour paste is added. Serve steak, spinach, rings of onions and wine sauce with roast potatoes.

TUSCAN BEAN STEW

Italy Taste: Tuscan Stew Bean

- 1 tbsp of olive oil extra virgin

- 50g of red onion, 30 g finely cut carrot, 30 g of celery finely chopped, finely cut

- One clove of garlic, finely cut.-

- 1 tsp of Provence herbs 200ml plant pot.

- Tomatoes 1 x 400 g chopped

- 200g of mixed beans

- 50g of freshly chopped Kale

- 1 tbsp of chopped Parsley

- 40g of buckwheat

Instruction:

1. Heat oil and fry the onion, carrot, celery, garlic, and grass in a cup of low to medium heat gently until vegetable soft.

2. Stir in the tomato puree with the stock. Attach the breasts and prepare for thirty minutes. Put the Kale and let it cook until smooth, then attach the Parsley for another 5-10 minutes.

3. Cook the buckwheat, drain and serve as required by packet instructions.

Reasons to Add Buckwheat

This is one of the suggested Sirtfoods food lists. Buckwheat is deceptive as it is entirely not synonymous with wheat. Buckwheat, in reality, is not a real grain but the fruit of a leafy plant in the same family as sorrel and rhubarb. It is often called pseudo-cereal because the grain is similar to cereal grains. The name Buckwheat comes from the Dutch word "buckwheat," most likely related to the vine's triangular fruits, which look like beechnuts. The buckwheat flour used for pancakes, crepes, or Noodle (Japanese soba) is most well-known to us in many cases.

There are ten reasons for trying the Sirtfood buckwheat: There are well-researched reasons:

1. The fiber of buckwheat is high and suitable for constipated persons.

2. The buckwheat protein has all nine essential amino acids (which are not produced by the body), making it closer to being "full."

3. It is necessary for tissue growth and repair with amino acid lysine.

4. This makes it suitable for those with wheat allergies, as sweetmeat is gluten-free.

5. It is rich with vitamins such as calcium, iron, vitamin E and B, magnesium, manganese, zinc, and copper.

6. Buckwheat magnesium helps to relax the vessels; it helps to improve circulation, reduces blood

pressure, and lowers cholesterol.

7. The blood sugar level is supported by buckwheat. This helps increase blood sugar levels evenly, due to the slower decomposition and absorption of carbohydrates in buckwheat. This is particularly good for those with diabetes by maintaining the blood sugar level.

8. It is also low in calories, which is useful for reducing the build-up of fat.

9. Buckwheat includes Sirtuin, a substance that strengthens capillary walls.

10. High in insoluble fiber, this Sirtfood helps women to avoid gallstones.

CHAPTER 5

SIRTFOOD DIET - WHAT ARE MEDJOOL DATES?

edjool Dates are tree fruits of the North-Africa and Middle-East region but are common in many desert-like areas all over the world. Dates usually constitute an essential part of Middle Eastern cuisine, while Medjool, even when dry, is especially appreciated for its large scale, sweet taste, and juicy meat. They have often eaten alone in a large meal or baking dish, as we mostly have in snacks or as a flavoring item.

The Discrepancy Between Other Forms of Dates

There are many specific times, although they all have some basic features. They are native to warm, arid climates, for example, on dated palm trees. Their fruit is new but most often dry, increasing its existence and avoiding spoilage at an early point. Medjools are generally considered to be "the highest" time. They are certainly the biggest and often the cost to purchase. Most consumers think their taste is also the best.

Medjools are informally referred to in their higher position as the "chief of dates," the "diamond of dates," or the "crown happiness of dates." It is what is considered a "sweet" day. Their texture and taste are usually categorized as soft, dry, or semi-dry. Soft dates are often called the most beautiful because it is so hard to grow and also because birds and insects are more susceptible to lose.

Taste Basics of Medjool Dates

The majority of people describe dates for Medjool as having a rich, almost caramel-like taste. Generally, they are served dried, although, in most situations, this drying is regular. The most common way to prepare some dates is to allow them, while still attached to the fruit, to maturate and sundry. Medjools do not need further treatment or care before serving when they are picked at the right time.

Nutritional Content

Just around 66 calories are in the dates of Medjool. It is a stable fiber source and includes significant amounts of needed minerals, such as potassium, magnesium, and copper. The bulk produces substantial fruit sugar so that it may be an excellent alternative to more calorie desserts. They are shared for nomadic travelers in the Middle East; there, they grow wild and provide a lot of healthy nutrients and energy that are also readily available to them.

How You Can Enjoy Medjool

However, one most comfortable way to enjoy dates is eating them alongside other finger foods such as crackers, hard cheeses, and crusty bread. The partners include a pit but are comprehensive and straightforward to clean in general.

The immense size of the fruit always fills as the pit is extracted. Walnuts, almonds, and wine are some of the more traditional things cooks should put in, but imagination is very spacious. To produce a unique flavor, certain people placed additional berries, tiny chocolate bits, or seasonal meats to the pit cellar.

Medjool Date Use in Cooking

A variety of recipes are even Medjool dates. Most North African stews, for example, call for sliced Medjools, which are typically combined in places such as Iran and Iraq with yogurt for breakfast. A variety of meat dishes are applied to flavor, which may also be mixed into the batter of different loaves of bread and pastries.

Where did the Medjool Dates Grow?

Palm date that is indigenous to North Africa and the Arab Peninsula is known to be Medjool-born. Fossil proof indicates that in countries as far as Saudi Arabia and Morocco, the fruits were enjoyed by older men, and their land is now the primary growing region in those nations. But, as with some people in Australia, other California growers had trouble raising the plants. They are often much harder to produce than other dates because they are sensitive to air quality and soil moisture. They usually take much energy and work to increase their demand, which is part of their relatively high price.

Cultivating Medjool Dates at Home

The fundamental way to grow a date palm from Medjool, though this is also the most time consuming and possibly stressful route, is by planting a pit and awaiting the germination. It can take twenty years for a sprouting tree to grow a productive crop. Home gardeners wishing to use Medjools for cultivation are generally better suited by buying proven plants from nurseries or nearby vendors or grafting branches onto new plants from existing palms. Trees usually take great care and maintenance for sunshine and soil quality to survive. Few gardeners managed to grow the plant's indoor greenhouses, but the best fruits are typically from trees in more natural conditions outside.

MATCHA GREEN TEA: A SIRT FOOD SUPERFOOD

What is Matcha?

This is simply pronounced as MA-cha, since the 12th century, it's been part of Japanese culture. It's one of Japan's most expensive drinks. Because of how the leaves have been formed, Matcha green tea differs totally from the regular green tea. Both teams come from the same mother plant named *Camellia sinensis*, a China-born shrub. This shrub brings about all sorts of tea leaves, such as black, green oolong, and white tea. Such drinks differ in their antioxidant content, caffeine content, and other nutritional properties depending on the region and how they are prepared.

What is the difference between Matcha and regular green tea?

Matcha is a special kind of tea much less refined than usual green tea as the leaves are never heated and kept shaded to protect the natural nutrients in the plants. Regular green tea is grown much more during processing and is dried in the sun, similar to the shade of Matcha. Matcha green tea is a bright green power which, instead of boiling and brewing methods used to produce traditional green tea, has also been dissolved in warm liquid. You often take a higher nutritional amount because you eat the whole leaves in a milder Matcha powder than tossing their leaves in a teabag as you do for a healthy tea.

How do you like Matcha?

Matcha has mildly green colors, but a more profound

and almost buttery scent. Like any green tea. It is particularly delicious mixed with a little extract of vanilla, some non-dairy milk, and stevia.

Matcha Superfood advantages:

• Far out of all the powerful super aliments we know about today, is Matcha green tea. Matcha contains more than 6-times the amount of antioxidants in Goji fruit, 7-times the number of antioxidants in dark chocolate, and 17 times the number of antioxidants in spinach. And it's only one tea cubicle!

• This is 137 times more commonly contained in daily green tea as a prominent antioxidant EGCG. EGCG is a part of the catechin-like antioxidant family that is related to improved heart function, proper metabolism, and healthier aging.

• The Matcha is a perfect way to enhance preparation as it's relaxing and anti-inflammatory.

• A lovely, vibrant, and green tea was also discovered to deter cancer as tea antioxidants are so potent that they help inhibit parasites of the immune system called free radicals.

• Five times more than standard tea for Matcha in chlorophyll. The green dye in plants that can support clean skin, preserve the heart and blood, and reduce joint inflammation is chlorophyll. This is often present in animals.

• A bottle of the Matcha tea is equivalent to 10 cups of standard green tea for fuel.

• A long stream of energy against a crash you get with caffeine, and perhaps help with weight control, was found to raise metabolism. Matcha is no substitution for an unsafe diet, but it's a much more intelligent, balanced way to improve and obtain strength.

• Terra Matcha also decreases the fear in Matcha because of the high raw concentrations of L-theanine. An L-theanine-an amino acid promotes relaxation, which is why regular green tea is regarded as a soothing drink.

• Matcha produces just 35 milligrams of caffeine per tablespoon, less than a cup of black coffee, almost one percent.

• Sounds impressive to a tea, isn't it? This is because Matcha has unique properties, like all plants, that make it very special. Mind that Matcha is not a magic pill that fixes quickly to full safety, but that it beats other teas and is a cheaper and less detailed choice.

Enjoy the green tea of Matcha:

Traditional-use: This tea can be enjoyed in the same way that you use green tea regularly. Boil in your favorite mug with a cup and a half of water and let it boil for 3-5 minutes. Gently put the Matcha green tea powder into 1/2 teaspoon. You will notice that it starts to spray a bit, which is natural. You may even apply a little un-dairy milk that gives it a more smooth flavor if you prefer. Or combine it all in your blender to make it frothier like drinks in the café.

Other uses: In a green smoothie, Matcha is always significant. You may use it to replace a pinch for the usual green superfood powder or to include it in some other daily smoothie. Because the Diet is so high, you don't need so much to benefit your health. Half to a whole tea cubicle is plenty.

In energy doughs, vegan ice creams, truffles, or even brownies and cupcakes, you can also use Matcha. Make it simple and blend it to an iced Matcha latte with some ice and non-dairy milk. Make yourself creative and see what you can do with Matcha.

Where to find and how to find Matcha:

No old Matcha tea brand is essential to purchasing. Many of the consumer labels of Matcha tea are not real, Matcha. The best products you see in the store are marginally cheaper than those in the inferior models, which means a superior price. For any Matcha you are buying, test the name. It will only have 100% Matcha green tea. It should be organic and ceremonial, implying that it is developed using the same limited green tea process used in Japan that does not include pesticides.

The color should also be bright green, not a dumb greenish-brown color indicating that the Matcha is more substantial or cheaper.

Most Matcha is sold in containers of 2-4 ounces, ranging from $15.00 to $50.00. These are certainly not cheap but will last for at least three months if you use a half tea cubicle per day.

GREEN JUICE-SIRT FOOD DIET

A significant component of this Diet is green tea. It is included in the recipes chapter, so we thought that it would be helpful to add it separately. The juice is full of nutrients and a great add-on to a regular diet, even if you don't intend to follow the Diet. However, it is essential to note that we have researched carefully that in a juicer, NOT in a mixer or a nutritional bull, a food processor, or whatever other than a juicer is necessary). We tested both approaches and can say that the mixed variety is a bad sweet flavor, that it is a reasonably tasty drink!

The green juice remains in the refrigerator for three days, so a whole deal to save time is worth producing. To save time in the morning, we usually make it just the night before. This green Sirtfood Diet is filled with rich Sirtfoods that are perfect for those who want a little health boost and essential for everyone adopting the Sirtfood Diet.

Ingredients:

- 30g of rocket

- 75g of kale

- Two celery sticks

- 5g of parsley

- 1cm of ginger

- ¼ green apple

- ½ lemon juice

- ½ tsp of Matcha green tea

Method

1. Juice all ingredients except lemon and green Matcha tea.

2. Hand in the soft green squeeze the lemon juice.

3. Put a little green liquid in a glass and mix the Matcha. In the glass, add the remaining green sauce and mix again.

4. Drink instantly or save later.

CHAPTER 6
KETO DIET AND SIRTFOOD DIET

L et's get real. How can the human body have so many different ways of slimming it down?

There seems to be another new diet every year, which comes in the hot press with the approval of some great celebrities. It makes its big debut and thanks to every popular magazine on the check-out line in the food store. Another health expert who is part of a popular lecture show explains the science behind this new diet as if it were an entire discovery.

Nevertheless, you cannot help but wonder if this may be the trick to help you get back into your favorite jeans long before the children are born. Or at least before adulthood, sorry sweetheart said your days are over to eat whatever you want without getting a single pound.

There have been two diet plans over the last few years that have brought it to the fore. The low-carbon, fatty

Keto diet and the "skinny gene" boost Sirtfood diet are available.

Hold up

What's the distinction between the two? What's best for your plans for health and weight loss? What is a "skinny gene" in the world?!

However, let us explore everything there is to know about each diet to answer your questions. This is your ultimate guide to everything behind them, the Sirt and the science.

What's the Keto Diet?

Let's continue with the diet keto, or ketogenic. In brief, a keto diet consists of a small consumption of starch, milk protein, and high-fat products. Real Keto peeps try to drink 20g or less of carbohydrates daily, most of which are consumed from healthy fat sources.

Invented by Peter Huttenlocher back in the 1970s, the notion behind this is that our body is in a state of ketosis. What now? What now? This is another excellent way to say that your metabolism does not rely on glycogen and begins to relish fat for energy.

Your body (especially your liver) releases small molecules called ketones that act to offer your body energy. At the same time, our sugar levels are somewhat low if you reduce your carb and calorie intake.

Ketones are made from fat, so your body is reprogrammed to fat in contrast to glucose on this diet. By limiting your calorie consumption and, in some ways, exerting your body to relish fat for fuel, fat stores are accessible throughout your body when you need energy.

Looks reasonable, okay? Now, we're going to switch gears and talk SIRT!

What's Sirtfood Diet?

Before we know about the SIRT diet program, let us be mindful of the fact that this diet allows you to consume (in moderation) red wine and chocolate. How can that be?

This latest diet plan, established by nutritionists, means that many Sirt products are eaten. This means foods that produce a protein called Sirtuin in our body.

These particular small proteins help reduce inflammation and defend our cells against stress damage. Ah, so sirtuins are for cells as we have red wine.

Everything's making sense!

Seriously, a Sirtfood diet will boost your metabolism and burn fat quickly. Men and women reported falling up to seven pounds a week after this diet plan had begun.

In contrast to the ketogenic diet, the diet is divided into two phases. You need to minimize your daily consumption to 1000-calories during the first three days while you have three green shirts- food juices plus one sirt-food meal daily.

Four to seven days, you can maximize your consumption to 1,500-calories while you enjoy 2-3 green juices and a Sirt meal a day. Then the next two weeks will be called the maintenance period, and your body will appear to be continuously losing weight.

This cycle is known to turn on a "skinny gene" when the body's healthy supply of energy is small by calories. However, there are few studies behind sort food. Research is still needed to understand Sirtuin and its effect on our healthfully.

That said, the sirt food diet produces big waves, and people around the world see results. Celebrities like pop singer Adele, who lost almost 50 pounds of SIRT food, show this program of weight loss combined with exercise works well. Sounds doable ... *a glass of wine *.

Keto Diet: What Can You Eat

And now that part you were all waiting for ... what you can eat! A keto diet consists of lots of high-fat foods, which are probably already in your fridge.

Seafood All vitamin-rich and keto-friendly, including Salmon, shrimp, halibut ... Be careful about specific types of shellfish, including palms, mustards, potatoes, and oysters, as high in carbs.

- **Low-carb vegetables**

Eat enough, greens! Such as Brussels, broccoli, and asparagus are nutrient-dense veggies that the ketogenic diet can eat in abundance. The list continues. However, it's a keto-friendly veggie as far it has a low-carbohydrate count.

- **Cheese**

Some of you say, Hallelujah! Yes, because it contains high-fat content, cheese is allowed in the keto diet. The best options are the mozzarella and cheddar cheeses. Be mindful of processed cheese and other high-sugar dairy products.

- **Avocados**

The California "delicacy" is a thing to enjoy on the keto diet. Avocado is high in fatty acids and omega 3. Great when mixed with some vegetables in a smoothie or a meal and equally great as a snack.

- **Poultry and Meat**

This is a staple of the keto diet. It has zero sugars and is full of useful vitamins. Suitable for meats higher in fat, like ribeye steaks and chicken thighs.

- **Eggs**

Another great source of protein, omega-3-fatty acids, and essential nutrients are eggs to be eaten at breakfast or midday snacks.

- **Coconut oil**

If you don't learn, cocoa oil is an excellent substitute for other cooking oils because when burnt at these high temperatures, it is safer. You know, it's suitable for rubbing on sunburn as you bounce on the beach showing your new bikini body from the keto diet.

- **Greek Yogurt**

Another tasty choice, Greek yogurt for you to enjoy. It's nearly a dessert! Treat yourself! Treat yourself!

- **Cottage cheese**

Not only a way to get your fats in, but it also helps to lower inflammation and heal muscles.

Sirtfood Diet: What Should You Eat?

Now that the long list of tasty things you will appreciate on the keto-diet is satisfied (and probably surprised), let's find out exactly what this mysterious "Sirtfood" is going and do it so that we will equate the two diet strategies.

- **Green Tea**

This is a critical component of a Sirtfood diet, and green tea consists of an essential bioactive Sirtuin called catechin, which decreases oxidative stress and accelerates metabolism. This acts as an appetite suppressant and picks me up beautifully. The better you do!

- **Medjool Dates**

Encouraged on diets of Sirtfood, Medjool dates are different from other periods because of the taste and texture they look like caramels. They have lots of health advantages, and they are trendy during this diet. They go well in the smoothie, and they are also better eaten as snacks to please your mouth. They also give excellent alternative tea or coffee sweetener.

- **Chocolate (must contain cocoa of at least 85%)**

To eat a small quantity of dark chocolate in the Sirtfood Diet without thinking about it! Only make sure that the cocoa content is at least 85% or higher.

- **Apples**

I know what they say. You know what they say. Eating an apple a day holds the doctor away, and an apple a day helps to prevent weight gain.

- **Tropical Fruits**

And we realize that citrus fruit is low in minerals, antioxidants, and carbohydrates, but now we learn that it is abundant in polyphenol and that it allows our bodies to lose fat and lean.

- **Parsley**

There are tons of antioxidants and minerals in this minty leaf. It supports bone safety and protects your view. To include the nutritional advantages of parsley as a garnish or blend with other cooked vegetables.

- **Turmeric**

This is a welcome additive to this diet plan for a medicinal herb with anti-inflammatory effects. A dose of 500 to 2,000 milligrams- turmeric per day is healthy.

- **Kale**

Among the world's most rich nutrient crops, kale can be eaten abundantly on the Sirtfood diet. Discover it in a smoothie or as a salad.

- **Berries**

Blueberries are a delightful pleasure to indulge in this diet, Earth's flavor. They are also excellent for hydration and full of vitamins.

- **Capers**

I bet that you did not realize the capers are an incredibly useful superfood. Caper can be used for diabetes, fungal infections, arthritis, and other conditions.

- **Red Wine**

Furthermore, red wine with open arms is accepted on a Sirtfood diet (in moderation, of course). They aren't the only recipes you should appreciate. Others include coffee, arugula, chilies, walnuts, etc. But you get the spit!

Keto Diet Benefits vs. Sirtfood Diet Benefits

The two conventional diets tend to encourage you to consume a wide variety of items that you need to cut out with specific foods to reduce your loses. They deliver a much more practical and enjoyable menu than a claim, the diet for cod soup. The main problem now is: which is one of these two diets is better for you?

A Keto diet can assist you in losing weight and also boost your health. You will help to understand acne and increase the heart and brain's efficiency and reduce the chance of life-threatening illnesses, such as some cancers. This was also reported to help minimize convulsions of small children.

Studies have shown that you can adhere to your diet primarily with a ketogenic diet for the long term, but your wellbeing must add more carbs, such as vegetables, fruit, and beans.

On the other side, a Sirtfood diet was also selected as a means of quick weight loss. It can defend you from chronic diseases and has anti-aging capabilities. Whether or not you're rigid with this diet plan, including these nutrient - rich Sirt foods menu in your diet will improve your wellbeing.

Nonetheless, for several reasons, this lifestyle is not practical in the long term. The ultra-low-carb diet and low calorie may be dangerous, and more work is needed to determine the effect on our bodies.

Conclusively, it seems that the Keto diet and the Sirtfood diet have both positive and negative effects. The reality is that all significant dietary improvements are likely to help you shed weight, and these current, innovative plans are realistic choices when appropriately implemented.

The ultimate focus is both the keto and Sirtfood diets on nutrient-rich foods and the positive response in our bodies to a higher metabolism, reduced inflammation, and excess fat burning. Perhaps a combination of these two diets is the best of all worlds? We'll leave it to learn with some wellness authority.

If you have your own weight loss goals and want to try a new approach, lifestyle changes like the ketogenic or Sirt food diet are worth a shot. Some diet that makes dark chocolate, wine, or high-fat mozzarella cheese cannot be too challenging at the end of the day.

CHAPTER 7
SIRTFOOD DIET DELICIOUS RECIPES

When you're thinking about trying the Sirtfood diet, we 're here to lend you a hand, with different types of delicious recipes. In the previous chapter, the book explains a 7-day program to lose 7 pounds on average, so including Sirtfood in your diet will aid in making you more comfortable.

Best Sirtfood Diet Recipes

SIRT FOOD JUICE The Sirtfood Juice is a good start – so we have tossed into the recipe to continue as a bonus extra. The book recommends consuming three juices and adding one meal for the first three days, accompanied by two sauces for the next 4 Green juice.

Ingredients:

- 2 big handfuls or 75kg of kale

- A big handful or 30g Rocket

- A small or 5g flat-leaf parsley

- Small handful or 5g of lovage leaves (optional)

- Green Celery with 2–3 full stalks or 150g, including its leaves

- 1/2 green apple.

- 1/2 lemon juice

- 1/2 standard tsp green tea matcha.

Instructions:

Combine the greens (Kale, Rocket, Parsley, and lovage, if used) and apply water. In juicing leafy vegetables, we consider those juicers may vary in their output, and you can have to re-juice the residues before you move to other ingredients. The goal is to obtain approximately 50ml of juice from the greens.

Now you should juice the Celery and apple. You should cut the lemon and even bring it into the juicer, although we consider it much better to only place the lemon in the juice by hand. At this stage, you will have a minimum of around 250 ml of liquid, maybe a little more. Just if the sauce is cooked and you can serve, add the green tea.

Place a little juice into a bowl, add the Matcha and blend vigorously with a fork or tea cubicle. In your first two drinks, we only use Matcha because of its low amounts of caffeine (the same quality as a standard teacup). If drinking late, it can keep people sleeping. Once the Matcha has been drained, then pour the remainder of the drink.

Give it a finishing stroke, and the juice will be able to drink. Feel free to add flat water to your taste.

1.SIRT MUESLI

In case you want to make this in bulk the night before, just mix all the dry ingredients and lock it in an airtight jar. Then, you need to substitute the strawberries and milk the next day, and it 's good to go.

Ingredients:

- 20 g of flakes of Buckwheat

- 10 g soft wheat puffs

- 15 g of chocolate flakes or cocoa dried

- 40 g dates Medjool, sliced and pitted

- 15 g of walnuts, chopped off

- 10 g nibs of cocoa

- 100 g, hulled and chopped strawberries

- 100 g of regular Greek yogurt (or substitute vegan yogurt like soy or coconut)

Instructions:

Combine all of the above items (leave the fruits and milk out if not eaten immediately).

2.AROMATIC CHICKEN BREAST WITH RED ONIONS AND CHILI SALSA AND TOMATOES.

Ingredients:

- 120 g skinless chicken breast.

- 2 tsp turmeric ground

- 1/4 lemon juice

- 1 tbsp of virgin olive oil

- 50 g kale, sliced

- 20 g of diced red onion

- 1 tsp of fresh ginger minced

- 50 g of Buckwheat

- The salsa

- 130 g tomato (approximately 1)

- 1 chili bird's head, finely chopped.

- 1 tbsp, thinly chopped capers

- 5 g of Parsley, thinly chopped

- 1/4 lemon juice

Instructions:

1. Taking the eye out of the tomato for the salsa and cut it very finely, so that as much liquid as possible is retained. Mix the chili, capers, pink, and lemon juice. Mix. You might place everything in a mixer, yet the concluding result is somewhat different.

2. The oven heats up to 220oC / gas 7. In 1-tsp of turmeric, the lemon juice, and a little fat, marinate the chicken breast. Place in ovenproof frying pot for about 5–10mins, add the marinated chicken to it and cook for one or two minutes on each side, then move to the oven and make this for about 8–10 minutes or to cook it until it has cooled. Switch off the cooker, cover with foil and leave for 5 minutes before serving.

3. Then, boil the kale for 5 minutes in a steamer. After which fry the onions and the ginger in a small quantity of oil until soft. Add the kale and fry for another minute. Then, boil the Buckwheat with the remaining turmeric

teaspoon according to packet instructions. Serve together with rice, tomatoes, and salsa.

3.SIRT FOOD BITES

Ingredients:

- 120 g of Walnuts

- 30 g dark chocolate (85% cocoa solids), broken into pieces;

- 250 g dates of Medjool, pitted

- 1 tbsp paste of cocoa.

- 1 tbsp turmeric powder

- 1 tbsp of virgin olive oil

- 1 tbsp of vanilla extract 1 to 2 tbsp of tea.

Instructions:

1. Put the walnut and chocolate in a food processor and process it until it has a fine powder.

2. Put all other ingredients except water and mix until the ball forms a mixture. You may add the rain to stop it from being sticky, depending on

the consistency of the mix.

3. Shape the mixture into bites and cool in a tight container for at least 1 hour before consuming them with your mouth. You can roll some balls into a bit more cocoa or dried cocoa to achieve a different finish. They can hold in your fridge for up to 7 days.

4.ASIAN-KIN- PRAWN-STIR-FRY WITH NOODLES OF BUCKWHEAT

Ingredients:

- 150 g of raw king crevasses shelled, deveined

- 2 tsp tamari (if you don't avoid gluten, use soy sauce)

- 2 tsp of virgin olive oil

- 75 g soba (noodles of Buckwheat)

- 1 clove of garlic, thinly chopped

- 1 chili bird 's head, finely sliced.

- 1 tsp of new ginger finely minced

- 20 g of cut red onions.

- 40 g of chopped Celery

- 75 grams of green beans, sliced.

- 50 g spinach, sliced roughly

- 100ml of chicken stock

- g lovage or leaves of Celery

Instructions:

1. Over high heat, heat the frying pan, then cook the creams for 2–3 minutes in 1 tamari seabed and 1-tsp of oil. Upload the crevices to a tray. Wipe out the pan with paper from the oven because you can need it. Boil the noodles for 5-8 minutes as instructed in the packet in boiling water. Drain and reserve.

2. The olive oil is hot, fry garlic, chili, red onion, ginger, beans, Celery, and Kale for 2–3 minutes. Then, introduce the stock and boil and then add vegetable and boil until cooked, but still crunchy for 1 or 2 minutes.

3. Put the creams, pasta, lovage/celery leaves into the bowl, and then let it boil.

5.STRAWBERRY BUCKWHEAT

Ingredients:

- 50g of Buckwheat

- 1 tbsp turmeric ground

- 80 g of avocado

- 65g of tomato

- 20 g onion red

- 25 g dates of Medjool, pitted

- 1 tbsp of capers

- 30 g of Parsley

- 100 g of strawberries

- 1 tbsp of virgin olive oil

- 1/2 lemon juice

- 30 g of Rocket

Instructions:

1. Boil the Buckwheat with the turmeric, as indicated in the packet. Drain and keep cool on one side.

2. Chop the avocados, peppers, red onions, bandanas, caps, and Parsley finely. Then, blend it with the fresh Buckwheat. Slice the strawberries and mix the lemon juice and oil gently in the salad. Serve on a rocket bed.

6.TURMERIC CHICKEN & KALE SALAD WITH HONEY DRESSING

Notes: Prepare the salad in preparation for 10 minutes before eating. Chicken can be supplemented by lean meat, chopped creeks, or trout. Vegetarians can use chopped or cooked quinoa mushrooms.

Ingredients:

For the Chicken:

- 1 tsp of ghee

- 1/2 of red onion, diced

- 250-300 g of Chicken lean or meat thighs sliced

- 1 big clove of garlic, thinly diced

- 1 turmeric tablespoon powder

- 1-inch lime zest

- 1/2 lime juice

- 1/2 teaspoon of salt and potato.

To the salad:

- 6 stalks of broccolini or two bowls of broccoli.

- 2 pumpkins or cucumbers seeds (pepitas)

- 2 big kale leaves, cut off and cut off stems

- 1/2 prosecutor, diced.

- Fresh leaves of coriander, chopped

- Handful of fresh, chopped pink leaves

For the dressing:

- 3 cubicle lime juice

- 1 little garlic clove, finely diced or rubbed.

- 3 tablespoons (I have used one tablespoon of avocado oil

- 2 tablespoons of virgin olive oil;

- 1 raw teaspoon sweetheart

- 1/2 full-grain tablespoon of Dijon mustard.

- 1/2 tea cubicle sea salt and pepper.

Instructions:

1. Heat the ghee over medium-high heat in a small frying dish. Add onion and sauté for 4-5 minutes at medium heat until white. Add the chicken thin and garlic and brush it over medium-high heat for 2-3 minutes, then separate.

2. Add lime juice, turmeric, lime zest, pepper, salt, and simmer for another 3-4 minutes, stirring sometimes. Set aside the cooked thinness.

3. Boil small water in a small saucepan while the chicken is cooking. Cook broccolini for 2 minutes. Chop into 2-3 pieces under cold water.

4. Put the pumpkin seeds in the small pot and boil for 2 minutes over medium heat, stirring regularly to avoid burning. Season with a slight amount of salt. Set aside. Raw pumpkin seeds are also suitable for use.

5. In a salad bowl, place the chopped kale and pour over the dressing. Massage the dressing with your

hands. It softens the kale, like citrus juice for fish or beef carpaccio – it 'cooks' it somewhat.

6. Throw in the broccoli, chicken, pumpkin seeds, fresh herbs, and avocado slices.

7 CHICKEN KALE AND MISO DRESSING-SIRT FOOD WITH BUCKWHEAT

Ingredients:

For the Noodles:

- 2-3 pounds of kale leaves (roughly cut from the stem)

- Noodles of 150 g/ 5 oz

- 3-4 mushrooms, sliced

- 1 teaspoon of coconut oil or ghee

- 1 dark, small diced onion.

- 1 chicken breast of medium free-range, cut or diced.

- 1 long, thinly sliced red chili (seeds in or out depending on how hot you are)

- 2 big cloves of garlic, fine diced.

- Tamari sauce 2-3 tablespoons (gluten-free soy sauce)

For the Miso Dressing:

- 1 1/2 cubic meter fresh organic miso.

- 1 Kuchar tamari sauce.

- 1

- virgin olive oil spoon

- One tablespoon of citrus or lime juice

- One tea Kuchar (optional)

Instructions:

1. Bring to boil a small bowl of water. Add the kale and cook until slightly wilted for 1 minute. Remove and reserve the water but bring it back to the boil. Add the soba noodles and prepare as directed (usually around 5 minutes). Rinse and set aside under cold water.

2. While the shiitake mushrooms are browned on both hands, cook for 2-3 minutes in a little ghee or cocoa oil (approximately one teaspoon). Sea

salt sprinkles and set aside.

3. Heat coconut oil or ghee over medium-high heat in the same frying pan. Saute the onion and chili for 2-3 minutes, then add the pieces of chicken. Then, cook for about five minutes over medium heat, then add the garlic, tamari sauce, and a little water splash. Cook for an extra 2-3 minutes, mix until chicken is cooked.

4. Finally, add the noodles of kale and soba and cook the chicken up.

5. Mix miso dressing and pour over the noodles right at the end of cooking, so that you have all the helpful probiotics alive and working in the miso.

8.ASIAN KING PRAWN SIRT FOOD RECIPES AS BUCKWHEAT NOODLES

Ingredients:

- 150 g of raw robbery, deveined

- 2 tsp tamari (if you don't avoid gluten, you can use soy sauce)

- 2 tsp of extra virgin olive oil

- 75 g soba (noodles of Buckwheat)

- One clove of garlic, finely chopped

- 1 chili bird 's eye, finely chopped

- 1 tsp of fresh ginger finely chopped

- Sliced 20 g red onions

- 40 g of Celery, cut and sliced

- 75 g of green beans, cut

- 50 g kale, chopped roughly

- The stock of 100ml chicken

- 5 g of Celery or lovage

Instructions:

1. Heat a pot over high heat and cook creams for 2–3 minutes in one teaspoon of tamari and one teaspoon of oil. Transfer the creeping things to a plate. Wipe the saucepan with kitchen paper, as you will use it again.

2. Cook noodles for 5–8 minutes in boiling water or as directed. Drain and hold.

3. In the meantime, cook garlic, chili, and ginger, red onion, Celery, Beans, and Kalc with medium-high heat in the remaining oil for 2–3 minutes. Add the stock and boil, then cook until the vegetables are cooked, but still crunchy for one or two minutes.

4. Add the creams, noodles, and lovage and celery leaves to the saucepan, bring it back to a boil and serve.

9.SALMON SALAD BAKED MINT DRESSING-SIRT FOOD

Ingredients:

- One fillet of salmon (130 g)

- 40 g blended leaves of salad

- 40 g young leaves of spinach

- Two radishes, selected and sliced thinly

- Slice 5 cm or 50 g of cucumber, cut into pieces

- Two onions of season, trimmed and cut

- One small handful (10 g) of pets, chopped roughly

For the Dressing:

- 1 tsp of low-fat mayonnaise

- 1 tbsp yogurt

- 1 tbsp vinegar of rice

- Two mint leaves, thinly chopped

- Salt and black pepper freshly ground

Instructions:

1. Preheat the oven to 180 ° C (200 ° C).

2. Place the fillet on a baking tray and bake until cooked for 16–18 minutes. Take off the oven and set aside. The salmon in the salad is equally excellent hot or cold. Simply cook the skin side of your salmon and remove the salmon from the skin with a fish slice after cooking. When cooked, it should slide off easily.

3. Blend mayonnaise, yogurt, rice vinegar, mint leaves and salt, and pepper in a small bowl and leave to stand for a minimum of 5 minutes to allow developing flavors.

4. Set on a serving plate, the saucer, and spinach with the radishes, cucumber, spring onions, and Parsley. Flake the cooked salmon on the salad and dress it.

10. CHOC CHIP GRANOLA-SIRT FOOD

Breakfast chocolate! Be sure to serve you lots of SIRTs with a cup of green tea. If you prefer, rice malt syrup can be replaced by maple syrup.

Ingredients:

* 200 g of Jumbo oats

* 50 g of pecans chopped

* 3 tbsp of light olive oil

* 20 g of butter

* 1 slice of dark brown sugar

* Two slices of rice malt syrup

* 60 g Good quality of 60 g (70%) Chips of dark chocolate

Instructions:

1. Preheat the oven to 130 degrees C (140 degrees C / Gas 3). Line a big bakery with a silicone sheet or bakery bowl.

2. In a full tub, combine the oats and pecans. Heat the olive oil, butter, brown sugar, and rice malt

syrup gently in a small non-stick frying pan till the butter is melted, and the sugar and have dissolved. Do not permit boiling. Pour the syrup over the oats and whisk until the oats are thoroughly coated.

3. Spread the granola across the bakery tray and spread it into the corners. Let mixture clumps with spacing instead of even spreading. Bake 20 minutes in the oven until golden brown is tinted on the edges. Remove from the oven and cool completely on the tray.

4. Divide any larger lumps with your fingers on the tray and then mix in the chocolate chips. Grab the granola in the airtight bath or container. The granola will remain for a minimum of 2 weeks.

11.FRAGRANT ASIAN HOTPOT-SIRT FOOD

Ingredients:

- 1 tsp of mashed tomato

- Anise 1 star, crushed (or 1/4 tsp of ground anise)

- Small handful (10 g) pets, finely cut stalks

- Small handful (1Og) coriander, thinly cut stalks

- 1/2 lime juice

- The chicken stock of 500ml, fresh or one cube

- 1/2 carrot, diced and minced in matches

- Cut 50 g of broccoli into tiny florets

- 50 g beansprouts

- 100 g small tiger crevices

- 100 g company tofu, cut.

- 50 g rice noodles cooked as advised by the packet

- 50 g water chestnuts fried, drained

- 20 g steak ginger, diced

- 1 tbsp of good quality paste

Instruction:

1. Put in a big pot the tomato purée, the star anise, the peanuts, coriander stalks, lime juice, and the chicken water, and cook 10 minutes for a meal.

2. Attach the cabbage, broccoli, prawns, tofu, pasta, and water chestnuts and cook until broken. Stir the sushi ginger and miso paste from the sun.

3. Serve with Parsley and coriander leaves the ground.

12.LAMB BUTTERNUT SQUASH AND DATE-SIRT FOOD

Unbelievable warm Moroccan spices make this balanced tagine perfect for chilly autumn and winter evenings. For an extra health kick, serve with buckwheat!

Ingredients:

- Two tbs of olive oil.

- Sliced one red onion

- Ginger 2 cm, grated

- Three cloves of garlic, grated or smashed.

- One tablespoon flakes of chili (or taste)

- Two teaspoons of cumin.

- One piece of cinnamon

- Two teaspoons of turmeric ground

- 800 g fillet lamb neck, cut into 2 cm pieces

- 1/2 tea cubicle salt

- 100 g of Medjool dates, pitted and chopped

- 400 g of Tomatoes diced, plus half a can of

water

- 500 g squash of butternut, cut into cubes 1 cm

- Drained 400 g tin chickpeas

- Two fresh coriander teaspoons (plus garnish extra)

- Buckwheat, couscous or rice to be served

Instructions:

1. Preheat the 140C oven.

2. Drizzle about two olive oil tablespoons in a large, ovenproof casserole dish or cast-iron casserole. Also, add the sliced onion and cook for about 5 minutes on a gentle heat until the onion is softened but not brown.

3. Add rasped garlic, chilies, cumin, cinnamon, and turmeric. Stir well and cook with the lid for one more minute. Add water sprinkling if it gets too dry.

4. Next, add chunks of lamb. Add the salt, caked dates and tomatoes to cover the meat with onions and spices, plus about half a can of water (100-

200 ml).

5. Carry the tagine to the boil and place the cover on, and place 1 hour 15 minutes into your preheated oven.

6. Add chopped butternut squash and drained chickpeas thirty minutes before finishing the cooking time. Stir it all, place the lid back and return to the oven for the last 30 minutes.

7. Remove from the oven and mix in chopped coriander when tagine is finished. Serve with buckwheat, couscous, or basmati rice.

Remarks

If you are not equipped with an ovenproof copper or iron casserole, just cook the tagine in a regular cup before it is in the oven and switch it back to a weekly casserole dish before putting it in the oven. Add an extra 5 minutes to cook to allow the casserole dish to be heated besides.

13.PRAWN ARRABBIATA-SIRTFOOD

Ingredients:

- 125-150 g Fresh or baked crevasses (ideally king crevasses)
- 65 g Pasta Buckwheat
- 1 tbsp of virgin olive oil

For sauce of arrabbiata

- 40 g of onion, sliced.
- 1-clove of garlic, finely chopped
- 30 g Celery, smoothly cut
- 1 Chili bird's head, finely minced
- 1 tsp Dried herbs 1 tsp
- 1 tbsp virgin olive oil
- 2 tbsp of White wine (optional)
- 400 g Tinned tomatoes chopped
- 1 tbsp Petty chopped

Instructions:

1. Fry oil, garlic, dried herb, chili and celery in oil for 1-2 minutes over medium-low heat. Turn to medium heat, add a little bit of red wine and cook for 1-2 minutes. Add the tomatoes and allow the sauce to cook for 20-30 minutes over medium-low heat till It's done and creamy consistency. Just add water in case you feel the sauce is too thick.

2. During the cooking process, a pan of water will be brought to the boil and pasta will be cooked as directed on the packet. Drain, mix with the olive oil when you are finished, and hold in the pot until appropriate.

3. When using raw prawns, add to the sauce and cook 3–4 minutes longer until they are opaque and pink, add the parsley and serve. If you use fried creeping pickles, add the sauce and allow it to boil and serve.

4. Gently add the parboiled pasta to the sauce and blend it, but do it gently and serve!

14.TURMERIC BAKED SALMON-SIRT FOOD

Ingredients:

- 125-150 g Salmon Skinned

- 1 tsp of virgin olive oil

- 1 tsp of turmeric field

- 1/4 Lemon juice

For the spicy celery:

- 1 tsp of Super virgin olive oil

- 40 g of onion, sliced.

- 60 g of red tinned lenses

- 1-clove of garlic, diced

- Fresh ginger, thinly cut

- 1 Chili eye of a bird, finely chopped

- 150 g of celery, then cut it in lengths of 2 cm

- 1 tsp Curry powder Moderate

- 130 g of tomato, cut into eight wedges

- 100 ml of chicken stock or vegetable stock

- 1 tbsp Petty chopped

Instructions:

1. Preheat the oven to a level of 200C / gas 6.

2. Continue with the celery spicy. Heat a pan over medium to low temperatures, add olive oil, then onion, garlic, ginger, chilies, and celery. Fry gently for about 3-4 minutes until it is soft and not brown, then apply the curry powder, then continue cooking for an extra minute.

3. Tomatoes and lentils should be added and gently cooked for 10 minutes. However, you might want the cooking time to be increased or decreased based on how crunchy the celery is.

4. In the meantime, rub over the salmon and mix oil, turmeric, and lemon juice. Cook in the bakery for 8–10 minutes.

5. Slice the parsley and the celery and serve with the salmon to end.

15.CORONATION CHICK SALAD-SIRT FOOD

Ingredients:

- 75 g of real yogurt

- 1/4 of a lemon juice

- 1 tsp Coriander, split

- 1 tsp of turmeric ground

- 1/2 tsp Curry powder Moderate

- 100 g Cooked chicken breast, cut into small pieces

- six halves of walnut, finely chopped

- 1 Date of Medjool, finely chopped

- 20 g Red onion, diced.

- 1 Chili with Bird's Eye

- Serve with 40 g Rocket

Instruction:

In a mug, add milk, lemon juice, coriander, and spices. Remove all the other components and put on a rocket table.

16. POTATOES BAKED WITH SPICY CHICKPEA STEW-SIRT FOOD

Mexican Mole Kind

North-African-Tagine, this Spicy Chickpea Stew is incredibly tasty and is an excellent topping point for baked potatoes with veggie, organic, gluten-free, and milk-free. And there's candy in it.

Ingredients:

- Pickled all over 4-6 baked potatoes

- two cucharks of olive oil.

- two red onions, thinly sliced

- four garlic leaves, dried or minced

- Ginger 2 cm, grated

- Chili flakes 1/2-2 teaspoons (depending on the hotness)

- Two cubs of cumin seeds

- Two turmeric teaspoons

- Heat spray

- Tomatoes 2 x 400 g tins

- two unsweetened cocoa powder teaspoons (or cacao)

- Two x 400 g tins of chickpeas (or, if you choose, kidney beans), plus water from Chickpeas NOT DRAIN!!!

- Split into bitesize bits 2 yellow peppers (or whatever hue you prefer!).

- two additional parsley teaspoons for garnish

- Salt and pepper (optional) to match

- Side salad (optional)

Instructions:

1. Heat the oven to 200C, while all supplies can be packed.

2. Put the sliced potatoes in the oven when the oven is high enough and cook for 1-hour or cook until they are soft like you.

3. Pour the olive oil and sliced the onion in a saucepan once the potatoes are in the oven and cook softly on with

a cover for 5-minutes until the onions are soft and tender, but not brown.

4. Remove the cap with garlic, ginger, chili, and cumin. Add the turmeric and a little water, then boil for extra 1-2 minutes, be careful, and do not let the pan get too dry.

5. Next, apply cocoa powder (or cacao) and chickpeas (even chickpea water) to pepper and tomatoes. Allow it to boil and simmer for 45-minutes on low heat until the sauce is thick and greasy (do not cause it to burn!). The stew will be made roughly at the same time as the potatoes.

6. Eventually, add two tablespoons of parsley and some salt and pepper if you want and serve the stew with a plain side salad on top of the baked potato, maybe.

17. GRAPE AND MELON JUICE-SIRT FOOD

Ingredients:

- 1/2 washed, halved, added and finely cut seeds if desired

- 30 g young leaves of spinach, stalks cut

- 100 g red grapes seedless

- 100 g of melon cantaloupe, peeled and cut into small pieces

Instructions:

In a juicer or mixer, blend until smooth.

18. KALE AND RED ONION DHAL WITH BUCKWHEAT-SIRT FOOD

Kale and Red Onion Dhal with Buckwheat are tasty and highly nutritious, fast, and easy to make, naturally gluten-free, milky, vegetarian, and vegan.

Ingredients:

- 1 tbsp of olive virgin oil

- 1-tiny sliced red onion

- three cloves of garlic, grated or crushed

- Ginger 2 cm, grated

- one chili, deserted, fine-cut birds of the eye (more if you like hot things!)

- 2 tbsp of turmeric

- Two tea cubs garam masala

- 160 g lentils

- 400ml of chocolate milk

- 200ml of water

- 100 g kale (or an excellent alternative for spinach)

- 160 g (or brown rice) buckwheat

Instructions:

1. In a big, deep saucepan, pour a little quantity of olive oil, then add the sliced red onion. Cook on medium heat, and make sure the cover is closed for 5 minutes.

2. Remove garlic, chili, and ginger and simmer for 1 minute longer.

3. Add water and turmeric to the garam masala and simmer for another 1 minute.

4. Add red lentils and 200 ml of milk (coconut) and water (just by half the cocoon milk can be filled with water and tipped into the pot).

5. Mix all together thoroughly and cook on a gently warm plate for 15-20 minutes. Extract and apply a little more water when the dhal starts to adhere.

6. After 20 minutes, introduce the kale, stir thoroughly and replace the lid, and you can then cook for another 5-7 minutes (1-2 minutes if instead of using spinach).

7. Place buckwheat in the medium saucepan for about 10-15 minutes, and you can do this before the curry is ready and add lots of boiling water. Make the water boil and then cook for an extra 10-minutes or more in case you want your buckwheat softer. Serve with you can dry the buckwheat in a sieve.

19. BEEF FOR WITH A RED WINE JUS, ONION RING, KALE AND ROASTED POTATOES-SIRT FOOD

Ingredients:

- 100 g, sliced and 2 cm diced potatoes
- 1 tbsp of virgin-olive-oil
- 5g sweet sliced parsley
- 50 g red onion, rings sliced
- 50 g of Sliced kale
- 1-clove of garlic, finely chopped
- 120–150 g or 3,5 cm fillet beef steak
- 40 ml of red wine
- 150ml of reserve beef
- 1 tsp of mashed tomato
- Dissolved 1 tsp of corn-flour in 1 tbsp of water

Instructions:

1. Oven power to 220oC / gas 7.

2. Put the peeled potatoes into a big pot of boiling

water, bringing it to boil and steam for 4–5 minutes, then rinse. Put in an oven a frying pan with one tablespoon and fry for 30–40 minutes in a hot oven. Change the potatoes every 8-10 minutes to make sure it is evenly cooked.

3.	Fry the onion over medium heat for 5-7 minutes in 1-teaspoon of oil until soft and well caramelized. Steam the kale for about 2-3 minutes then drink. Cook the garlic softly in a ½-teaspoon of oil for 1-2 minutes until it is soft and not colored.

4.	Cook the meat in a tablespoon of the oil and fried in an ovenproof pot over medium to high heat according to how you want the meat to be cooked. In case you want the meat to be medium, it is better to turn the meat and then move the pot to the oven set at 220 ° C / gas seven and finish the cooking for specified times.

5.	Take the meat out of the container and put back to cool. Put the wine in the hot-bowl and absorb the traces of beef. Bubble until the wine is full, syrupy, and condensed.

6.	Add stock and tomato puree to the steak and simmer and then apply the paste with maize flour to thicken the sauce and add until you have the desired consistency for a little more time. Mix this with any steak juice and combine with the potatoes roast, kale, onion circles, butter, and red wine.

20 BLACKCURRANT AND KALE SMOOTHIE-SIRT FOOD

Ingredients:

- 2 tsp honey

- 1 cup of freshly made green tea

- 10 kale baby seeds, cut stalks

- 1 fully ripe banana

- 40 g blackcurrants, cleaned and cut stalks

- six blocks of ice

Instructions:

1. Mix the honey in warm green tea, then whisk all the ingredients together into a mixer until smooth. Drink straight away.

21.BUCKWHEAT PASTA SALAD-SIRT FOOD

Ingredients:

- 50 g Buckwheat Pasta (cooked as instructed by packet)

- Big handful of rockets

- Small handful of basil leaves

- eight cherry tomatoes (halved)

- 1/2 avocado, sliced

- 10 olives

- 1 tbsp of virgin-olive-oil

- 20 g pine nuts

Instruction:

1. In a small container, mix all the ingredients except the pine nuts and put them over the top on a plate or bowl.

22 GREEK SALAD-SIRT FOOD

Ingredients:

- Two wooden skewers

- Eight big black olives

- Eight tomatoes of cherry

- One yellow pepper, eight squares sliced

- 1/2 red onion, halved and divided into eight pieces

- 100 g (approximately 10 cm) of cucumber, cut into four parts and halved

- Cut 100 g feta into 8-cubes

For the dressing:

- 1/2 lemon juice

- 1 tbsp of virgin-olive-oil

- 1 tsp of Vinegar Balsamic

- 1/2 garlic clove, peeling and crushed

- Few leaves of basil, finely chopped (or 1/2 tsp of dry mixed herbs for basil and oregano substitution)

- Few oregano leaves, finely chopped

- A right blend with black pepper and salt

Instruction:

2. Thread each skewer in a sequence of salad ingredients: olive, tomato, yellow pepper, red ointment, cucumber, tomato, olive, pepper yellow, onion red, cucumber, and feta.

3. In a small bowl, place all the dressing ingredients and mix them thoroughly together. Pour over skewers. Pour over skewers.

23.KALE, EDAMAME AD TOFU CURRY-SIRT FOOD

A warm, windy curry. Easy to keep for another day cool or frozen.

Ingredients:

- 1 tbsp of rape oil

- one big onion, cut

- four garlic leaves, peeling and brushing

- one broad thumb (7 cm) fresh, peeled and broken ginger

- one red, desired, thinly sliced chili

- 1/2 tsp turmeric ground

- 1/4 tsp Cayenne pepper

- 1 tsp of peppers

- 1/2 tsp cumin ground

- 1 tsp of salt.

- 250 g red dried lenses

- 1 liter of boiling water

- 50 g of frozen soybeans

- 200 g of solid tofu, sliced into cubes

- Two tomatoes, chopped roughly

- One lime juice

- 200 g of kale leaves, torn stalks

Instructions:

1. In a frying pan, pour the oil and heat over medium heat. Put the onion, then fry the onion

for about 5-minutes before putting the garlic, ginger, and chili. Stir in the turmeric, cayenne, onions, cumin, and oil. Remove and stir again before adding the red lentils.

2. Pour into boiling water, then cook for another 20-30 minutes, till the curry has formed a thick puree.

3. Add the tofu, tomatoes, and soya beans. Then, cook for about 5-minute or more. Add the lime juice, kale and boil until the kale is soft.

24. CHOCOLATE CUPCAKES MATCHA ICING-SIRT FOOD

Ingredients:

- 150 g self-rearing meal

- 200 g sugar caster

- 50 g of cocoa

- 1/2 tsp of salt

- ½ of Fine espresso coffee decaf if preferred

- 120 ml of dairy

- 1/2 tsp of vanilla extract

- 50 ml of vegetable oil

- One egg

- 120 ml of boiling water

For the refrigeration:

- 50g of butter at room temperature

- 50 g of sweet coating

- 1 tbsp green tea powder

- 1/2 tsp of vanilla bean paste

- 50 g of soft cream

Instructions:

1. Preheat oven to a fan of 180C/160C. Cover the cake with a cupcake tray.

2. Put flour, sugar, cacao, salt, and espresso powder and thoroughly mix in a large bowl.

3. To dry ingredients, add vanilla extract, milk, egg, and vegetable oil, then use an electric mixer to blend well together. Pout hot water

gently and mix until it is well mixed. Use high speed to add air to the batter for another minute. The mixture has too much oil than a regular mixture of cake. Have confidence, and it's going to taste amazing!

4. Spoon the batter uniformly among the cake cases. No more than 3⁄4 full should be available for each cake case. Bake 15-18 minutes in the oven until the mixture gets bounced back. Make sure you remove it from the oven and then allow it to cool down and apply full icing.

5. To make the icing together, make the butter and the icing sugar pale and smooth. Attach the mixture of Matcha and vanilla and blend again. Then add cream cheese and beat to smooth. Pipe or sprinkle through the cakes.

25 SESAME CHICKEN SALAD-SIRT FOOD

Ingredients:

- 1 tbsp of sesame seeds

- One cucumber, peeled, half-long, teaspoon and diced,

- 100 g of baby kale, chopped roughly

- 60 g of pak choi, chopped finely

- 1/2 red onion, sliced very finely

- Wide handful (20 g) pets, hacked

- 150 g of chicken fried, shredded

For the Dressing:

- One lime juice

- 1 tbsp of virgin olive oil

- 1 tsp of his oil

- One lime juice

- 1 tsp transparent love

- 2 tsp of soy sauce

Instructions:

1. Sesame seeds are browned and fragrant in a hot saucepan for 2 minutes. Transfer to a cooling plate.

2. Mix the sesame oil, olive oil, honey, lime juice, and soy sauce in a small bowl.

3. Put the kale, cucumber, pak choi, red onion, and parsley and mix gently together in a large bowl. Put the dressing over and mix again.

4. Spread the salad of shredded chicken between two plates on the floor. Just before serving, sprinkle over the sesame seeds.

26 MUSHROOM SCRAMBLE EGGS SIRT FOOD

Ingredients:

- Two eggs

- 1 tsp soil turmeric

- 1 tsp of mild curry powder

- 20 g kale, chopped roughly

- 1 tsp of virgin olive oil extra.

- 1/2 chilly bird's eye, thinly sliced

- A handful of thinly sliced button mushrooms

- 5 g of parsley, perfectly chopped

- Set as a topper with seed mixture and spice any rooster sauce.

Instructions:

1. Mix curry powder and turmeric and add a small quantity of water until a light paste is obtained.

2. Then, you can steam the kale for about 2-3 minutes.

3. Over medium-high heat, heat the oil in a frying pan and fry the chili and mushrooms for 2-3 minutes until browned and softened.

27 CHICKEN BREAST WITH KALE, RED ONION AND SALSA-SIRT FOOD

Ingredients:

- 120 g chicken breast skinless

- 2 tsp soil turmeric

- ¼ of lemon juice

- One teaspoon of virgin-olive-oil

- 50 g of kale, cut

- Sliced 20 g red onion

- 1 tsp of fresh ginger chopped

- 50 g of buckwheat

Instructions:

1. Making the salsa, you need to remove the eye from the tomato then cut it finely, ensuring that the liquid is kept as much as possible. Capers, chilies, lemon juice, and parsley are all mixed.

You can put it all in a blender, but the end result is a little different.

2. Oven heat to 220oC / gas 7. Marinate in 1 teaspoon turmeric, lemon juice, and a small oil the chicken breast. Leave for five to ten minutes.

3. Heat a frying pan ovenproof till it is heated, add the chicken marinated and boil for 1-2 minutes on each side and then move it to the oven (place it on a bakery if the pot is not stove-proof) for about 8-10 minutes or until you have cooked it. Take it off the oven, ad cover it a thin foil, and allow it to cool for about 4-5 minutes serving.

4. However, cook the kale for 5 minutes in a steamer. Freeze the red onions and ginger in a small quantity of oil and add the cooked kale, then fry for another minute, until it is very soft and not brown.

5. Then, you can cook the buckwheat with the remainder of turmeric in accordance with the

packet instructions. Eat with rice, tomatoes, and salsa. Serve.

28.SMOKED SALMON OMELETTE-SIRT FOOD

You can try this easy and easy-to-cook recipe. It is full of goodness and flavor.

Ingredients:

- 2 small eggs

- 100 g of salmon smoked, sliced

- 1 tbsp of capcrs

- 10 g of the rocket, cut

- 1 tbsp of parsley, chopped

- 1 tbsp virgin-olive-oil

Instructions:

1. Crack the eggs and whisk them well in a bowl. Add salmon, cabins, rocket, and peregrinate.

2. Heat the non-stick frying pan and pour the olive oil until this is hot and not smoking. Add the egg mixture then transfer the mixture around the pan until it is even with a spatula or

fish slice. Reduce the heat and prepare the omelet. Glide the spatula around the sides and roll or flip half the omelet to eat.

29. GREEN TEA SMOOTHIE-SIRT FOOD

This super-healthy smoothie uses a highly concentrated green tea of Matcha powder. It is available in Asian specialists or tea shops.

Ingredients:

- Two big ripe bananas

- 250 ml of dairy milk

- 2 tsp of Matcha

- 1/2 tsp vanilla bean paste or a little scrape of vanilla pod seeds

- Six blocks of ice

- 2 tsp honey

Instruction:

1. Mix all ingredients in a mixer and drink in two containers.

30.MISO-MARINATED-COD with STIR-FRIED Greens & SESAME-SIRT FOOD

Ingredients:

- 20 g of Miso

- 1 tbsp of mirin

- 1 tbsp of virgin-olive-oil

- 200 g fillet of skinless cod

- Sliced 20 g red onion

- Sliced 40 g celery

- A clove of garlic, finely chopped

- One chili bird 's eye, finely chopped

- 1 tsp of fresh ginger finely chopped

- 60 g of green beans

- 50 g of spinach, sliced roughly

- 1 tsp of sesame seeds

- 5 g of parsley, chopped roughly

- 1 tbsp of Tamari

- 30 g of Buckwheat

- 1 tsp turmeric ground

Instructions:

1. Mix the miso, mirin, and one oil tea cubicle together. Rub the entire cod and leave for 30 minutes to marinate. To 220oC / gas seven fire the oven.Bake 10 minutes of cod.

2. Heat a big frying pan using the remainder of the oil. Remove cabbage, deep fry, then substitute celery, garlic, chili, ginger, green beans, then kale for few extra minutes. Fry until the kale is tender and cooked. Then, you may need to add a little water to the pot to help cook.

3. Then, you need to cook the buckwheat with turmeric for 3-5 minutes as directed on the packets.

4. Serve with the greens and serve in the stir-fry with the sesame beans, silk, and tamari.

31.RASPBERRY AND BLACKCURRANT JELLY-SIRT FOOD

Ingredients:

- Raspberries of 100 g, washed

- Two gelatin leaves

- 100 g of washed cassava

- 2 tbsp sugar granulated

- 300ml of water

Instructions:

1. Arrange in two glasses/ serving dishes/molds the raspberries. Leave the gelatinous leaves to soften in a bowl of cold water.

2. Stick in a small pot of sugar and 100 ml of water with the blackcurrants and let it boil. Allow it to simmer thoroughly, and then you can proceed to remove it from the heat for 3-5 minutes. Finally, Leave 2-3 minutes to stand.

3. Squeeze the gelatin leaves with excess water and add this gelatinous content to the casserole. Remove until completely dissolved,

then add to the remainder of the water. Put the liquid into the prepared dishes and cool. The jellies should be available in approximately 3-4 hours or overnight.

32.APPLE PANCAKES WITH BLACKCURRANT-SIRT FOOD

These pancakes are healthy but decadent. A perfect faint-hearted breakfast treat.

Ingredients:

- 75 g oats porridge

- 125 g flat meal

- 1 tsp powder baking

- 2 tbsp sugar caster

- Salt pinch

- 2 washed, cored apples and sliced into tiny parts

- 300ml of semi-skimmed milk

- egg-white

- 2 tsp of light olive oil

For the mixture:

- 120 g of blackcurrants, washed and removed stalks

- 2 tbsp sugar caster

- 3 tbsp of water

Instructions:

1 Make the compote first. In a small pan, put the sugar, blackcurrants, and water. Bring to a frying pan and cook 10-15 minutes.

2 Put oats, meal, baking powder, salt, and caster sugar and mix well in a large bowl. Mix the apple in and whisk for some time till it turns to the milk until you have a smooth blend. Sprinkle the egg whites to high tops, then insert onto the batter pancakes. Transfer to a jug the batter.

3 Heat about 1/2 tsp oil in a stockpot over medium-high heat, add around one-quarter of the batter. Fry until it is golden-brown on both sides. Repeat this process to make four pancakes.

4 You can then serve the blackcurrant compote

pancakes sprinkled.

33.FRUIT SALAD-SIRT FOOD RECIPES

This salad is packed with the best and essential Sirt fruit.

Ingredients:

- 1/2 cup of fresh green tea

- 1 tsp of honey

- One orange (halved)

- One potato, cored and diced roughly

- Ten red grapes without seed

- 10 of blueberries

Instructions:

1. Stir the sweetheart in half a mug of green tea. When dissolved, add half the orange juice. Let cool. Let cool.

2. Cut the remaining half of the orange and bring the mango, grapes, and blueberries together in a dish. Pour the cooled tea over and leave a few minutes before serving.

34. SIRT FOOD BITES RECIPES

Ingredients:

- 120 g of Walnuts

- 30 g of dark chocolate (85%cocoa solid), broken into pieces

- 250 g of Medjool, pitted

- Take 1 tbsp paste of cacao

- 1 tbsp of ground turmeric

- 1 tbsp of olive oil extra virgin

- 1 vanilla pod scraped seed or 1 tsp of vanilla extract

- Add 1-2 tbsp of water.

Instructions:

1. Place the walnuts and chocolate in a food processor and process until you have a fine ground powder.

2. Then, add all other ingredients with the exception of water and mix until a ball is made. Depending on the consistencies of the mix, you

can/not add water – you don't want it to be too sticky.

3. Form the mixture into small balls with your hands and cool in a close container for about 60 minutes before eating.

4. You could roll some of the balls to a different finish in some cocoa or desiccated cocoa if you want.

5. They can stay in your refrigerator for almost a week.

35.SIRT MUESLI RECIPES

Ingredients:

- 20 g of buckwheat puffs

- 10 g of buckwheat flakes

- 15 g of cocoa flakes or cocoa desiccated

- 40 g of Medjool pitted and chopped\

- 15 g of Walnuts, chopped

- 10 g of nibs of cocoa

- Hulled and chopped 100 g of strawberries

- 100 g plain Greek yogurt (or alternative vegan yogurt such as soy or cocoon)

Instructions:

1. Combine together all of the above ingredients and add yogurt and strawberries only before serving if made in bulk.

36.CHINESE-STYLE PORK PAK CHOI-SIRT FOOD

Ingredients:

- 400 g of tofu, cut into big cubes

- 1 tbsp of maize flour

- 1 tbsp of water

- 125ml of chicken stock

- 1 tbsp wine for rice

- 1 tbsp of pureed tomato.

- 1 tsp of sugar (brown)

- 1 piece of soy sauce

- 1 garlic clove, skinned and crushed

- 1 fresh ginger thumb (5 cm), peeling and rinding

1 tbsp of rapeseed oil

- Sliced 100 g shiitake mushrooms

- 1 shallot, peeling and slicing

- 200 g of Choi sum or pak choi, cut 400 g of thin pork (10 percent fat) into thin slices

- 100 grams of beansprouts

- A handful (20 g) of parsley, cut.

Instructions:

Upon kitchen paper lay tofu out, cover with more kitchen paper and reserve.

1. In a small bowl, mix corn-flour and water together, eliminating all the lumps. Stir in chicken potato, rice wine, puree of tomatoes, brown sugar, and soy sauce. Add the broken ginger and garlic and stir very well.

2. Heat oil at a high temperature in a wok or large frying pan. Add the Shiitake mushrooms and fry until cooked and sparkling for 2–3 minutes. Remove the pan with a slotted spoon from the mushrooms and set aside. Load the tofu in the

bowl and stir-fry on both sides until white. Take a slotted spoon and put aside.

3. Take the shallot and add the Choi to the wok, remove it for two minutes and add the thin. Cook until the thinner is ready, attach the sauce and reduce the heat for a little and bubble the sauce around the meat for one to two minutes. Attach the sprigs, shiitake champignons, and tofu to the bowl. Remove from heat, remove the parsley and serve as soon as possible.

37. TUSCAN BEAN STEW-SIRT FOOD

Ingredients:

- 1 tbsp of virgin-olive-oil

- 50 g of red onion finely cut.

- 30 g of carrot, finely chopped

- 30 g celery, finely cut and trimmed

- 1 garlic clove, neatly sliced.

- 21/2 of half bird's eye chili, finely sliced (optional)

- 1 tsp with herbs of Provence.

- Stock 200ml of vegetable

- Take 1 x 400 g of Italian chopped tomatoes

- 1 tsp of pureed tomato.

- Approximately 200 g tinned blended beans

- 50 g kale, sliced roughly

- Towering 1 tbsp poorly sliced parsley

- 40 g of buckwheat

Instructions:

1. Put the oil over low heat in a medium casserole and cook carrot, onion, celery, chili, garlic, and herbs gently until the onion is soft and not brown.

2. Connect the stock and the tomato puree to the simmer. Stir in the beans and let it simmer for about 25-30 minutes.

3. Add the pepper and let it cook for another 5–10 minutes. You can then add the parsley until tender.

4. Meanwhile, cook the buckwheat, dry, and

serve with the stew, as directed in the packet.

38.SALMON SIRT SUPER SALAD-SIRT FOOD

Ingredients:

- 50 g of rocket

- 50 g leaves of chicory

- 100 g of smoked salmon (lens, chicken breasts or tinned tunas may also be used)

- 80 g avocado, peeling, stoning and slicing

- Sliced 40 g celery

- Sliced 20 g red onion

- 15 g of sliced walnuts

- 1 tablespoon of capers

- 1 big Medjool date, pitted and chopped

- 1 tbs of olive oil extra-virgin

- 1/4 lemon juice

- 10 h of parsley, minced

- 10 g of lovage or celery leaves, split

Instructions:

1. Arrange the leaves of the salad on a large plate. Mix with all the other components and put on top of the plate.

NEW SIRTFOOF RECIPES

39 CHICKEN ESCALOPE WITH CAPER, SAGE AND PARSLEY, AND SWEET 'COUSCOUS' CAULIFLOWER

Ingredients:

- 150 g of cauliflower, chopped roughly

- 1 garlic clove, fine chopped

- 40 g of red onion, smoothly cut.

- 1 chili of the bird's eye, finely chopped

- 1tsp fresh, finely chopped ginger

- 2tbsp olive oil extra virgin

- 2tsp turmeric field

- 30 g Sun-dried, finely sliced tomatoes

- 10 g petroleum

- 150 g turkey scoping

- 1tsp smart dry

- 1/2 lemon juice

- 1 tablespoon capers

Instructions:

1. In a food processor, place the cauliflower and pulse in 2 seconds, chop it finely until they look like couscous. Set aside. Set aside. In 1 tsp of oil, cook the garlic, red onion, chili, and ginger until it is soft but not flavored. Attach turmeric and coolant and cook for 1 minute. Remove the heat and add tomatoes and half the parsley to the sun-dried tomatoes.

2. Cover the turkey in remaining oil and cook it for 5-6 minutes and change periodically. Attach the lemon juice, sleeping cats, capers, and 1 tbsp of water to the pan and eat.

40. GRANOLA-NEW SIRT FOOD CHOC CHIP

Breakfast cake! Make sure to bring you lots of SIRT with a cup of green tea. If you choose, rice malt syrup may be supplemented by maple syrup.

Ingredients:

- 200 g of Jumbo oats

- 50 g of pecans, chopped

- Medium or 3 tablespoons of olive oil

- 20 g of butter

- 1 tablespoon of dark brown sugar

- 2 strips of rice malt syrup

- High content of 60 g (70%)Chips with dark chocolate

Instructions:

1. Preheat oven to 160 ° C (Fan / Gas 3 at 140 ° C). Line a large bakery with a silicone layer or bakery.

2. In a large bowl, mix oats and pecans together. Heat olive oil, butter, brown sugar, and rice

malt syrup in a small non-stick pot till all the butter has melted, and the sugar and syrup are dissolved. Do not authorize boiling. Pour the syrup over the oats and whisk until the oats are completely covered.

3. Distribute the granola over the bakery, which spreads right in the corners. Having mixture clumps with spacing instead of distributed uniformly. Then, proceed to bake in an oven for 20 minutes until light brown slightly tinged on the outside. Make sure you remove the container from the oven and let it cool completely on the plate.

4. Separate the bigger lumps with your fingertips on the tray while cold and then mix in the chocolate chips. Place the granola or scoop into an airtight bath or container. Granola must stay for a minimum of 2 weeks.

41.THE BRAISED PUY LENTILS-NEW SIRT FOOD DIET

Ingredients:

- Halved 8 cherry tomatoes

- 2 tsp of extra virgin olive oil

- 40 g of red onion, sloping thinly

- 1 clove of garlic, thinly minced

- 40 g celery, cut thinly

- 40 g carrots, peeling and chopping thin

- 1 tsp of seasoning

- 1 tsp of thyme (dry or fresh)

- 75 g lentils

- 220 ml of stock of vegetables

- 50 g of spinach, sliced roughly

- 1 tbsp of parsley, diced

- 20 g of rocket

Instructions:

1. Heat up to 120oC / gas 1/2 of the oven.

2. In a small tin, place the tomatoes and roast in the oven for 35-45 minutes.

3. Cook a casserole over medium-low heat. Add one olive tablespoon with red onion, garlic, celery, and carrot and fry until soft for 1–2 minutes. Mix the paprika and thyme together and simmer for one more minute.

4. Rinse the lenses into a fine-tuned sieve and attach them with the stock to the bath. Let it boil, reduce the heat, and cook gently on the saucepan for 20 minutes. Add a little water after 7 minutes to the pan if the level drops too high.

5. Introduce the cabbage and cook for another 10 minutes. Stir in the parsley and rusty tomatoes when the lentils are baked. Serve with a rocket and the remaining olive oil teaspoon.

42. SHAKSHUKA-NEW SIRTFOOD DIET

Enjoy this spicy fried egg and kale healthy recipe

Ingredients:

- 1 tsp of extra virgin olive oil

- 40 g of red onion, finely cut

- 1 clove of garlic, thinly minced

- 30 g of celery, finely diced

- 1 Bird's eye chili, sliced thinly

- 1 tsp of cumin field

- 1 tsp of plant turmeric

- 1 tsp of seasoning

- 400 g Tinned Tomatoes Diced

- 30 g of kale, removed stems and chopped roughly

- 1 tbsp of parsley, chopped

- 2 small eggs

Instructions:

1. Heat a medium-low fire, thin, deep-sided frying pan. Add the oil and fry for 1 to 2 minutes with onion, garlic, celery, chili, and spices.

2. Add the tomatoes and then allow the sauce to slowly steam for 20 minutes, sometimes stirring.

3. Add the kale and cook 5 minutes longer. If the sauce is too thick, just add a little water. Stir in the parsley if your sauce has a nice rich flavor.

4. Make in the sauce two small wells and split each egg into them. Reduce heat to the lowest level and cover with a lid or foil the saucepan. Let the eggs cook for 10-12 minutes so that the white ones are firm while the yolks are still going. Cook for another 3-4 minutes if the yolks are tight. Serve right away – ideally straight from the saucepan.

43 VIETNAMESE TURMERIC FISH HERBS & MANGO SAUCE-NEW SIRT FOOD

Ingredients:

Fish:

- 1/4 lbs. new, monkeys, skinless cod, cut into 2 "long bits, approx. 1/2" thick

- 2 tbsp coconut oil (plus a few more tablespoon if required) for the fish pan-fry.

- Small marine pinch to taste

The marinade of fish: (Marinade for at least 1 hour or for overnight)

- 1 tbsp powder turmeric

- 1 teaspoon of salt

- 1 tbsp Chinese wine (Alt. dry sherry)

- 2 tsp small ginger

- 2 cubicles of olive oil.

scallion and Dill Oil infused:

- 2 cups of scallion (long-form slice)

- 2 fresh dill cups

- Sea salt shakes to compare.

Mango sauce dipping:

- 1 big mango rib

- 2 tbsp vinegar of rice

- 1/2 lime juice

- 1 clove of garlic

- 1 tsp dry red pepper chili (stir in before serving)

Toppings:

- Fresh coriander (whatever you like)

- Lime (as much as you want)

- Cashew nuts or pine nuts)

Instructions:

Steps:

1. Start by marinating the fish for at about 1 hour or overnight.

2. Place all ingredients in a food processor under "Mango dipping sauce" and mix until desired.

Pan-fry The Fish:

1. Heat 2-tbsp of coconut oil on high heat in a large non-stick bowl. Apply the pre-marinated fish when dry. * Note: Store the fish slices individually in the pot and, where required, separate them into two or more batches.

2. A loud sizzle, after which the heat can be decreased to medium-high, should be heard.

3. Do not switch the fish or push it until about 5 minutes you see a golden brown on the leg. Top with a pinch of salt from the sea. Add more coconut oil if necessary to fry the tuna.

4. When the fish is golden brown, turn the fish carefully to brush on the other side. Transfer to a large plate once it is done. * Note: In the frying pan, some oil will be included. The majority of the oil is used to create scallion and dill infused oil.

Infused-oil to make the scallion and dill:

1. In the frying pot, use the rest of the oil for medium to high heat, add 2-cups of scallions,

and 2 cups of dill. Turn off the heat after the scallions and dill have been added. Give them a gentle toss only about 15 seconds until the scallions and dill have faded. Spray with a splash of salt from the sea.

2. Pour over the fish the scallion, dill, and infused oil and serve with fresh cilantro mango dipping sauce, lime, and nuts.

44 MOROCCAN SPICED EGGS-NEW SIRT FOOD

Ingredients:

- 1 tsp olive oil

- 1 shallot, skinned and sliced

- 1 red pepper (bell), seeded and finely chopped

- 1 garlic clove, peeling and slicing thinly

- 1 courgette (zucchini), finely sliced and peeled

- 1 tbsp puree tomato (paste)

- 1/2 tsp mild powder chili.

- 1/4 tsp cinnamon ground

- 1/4 tsp of cumin ground

- 1⁄2 tsp. of salt

- 1 Tomatoes can be chopped up to 400 g (14 oz)

- Chickpeas can be 1 x 400 g (14 oz) in water.

- A little handful of petanque (10 g (1/3 oz)), chopped

- 4 room temperature medium eggs

Instructions:

1. Heat the oil in a cup, add the shallot and red pepper (bell) and fry gently for 5 minutes. Attach the garlic and courgette and simmer for another minute or two. Add the tomato puree, spices, and salt and stir.

2. Add the chopped tomatoes and the chickpeas to medium heat (soaking and all liquor). Cover the sauce with the cover and cook for 30 minutes-make sure it bubbles softly throughout and encourage it to diminish in volume by approximately one third.

3. Remove from the heat and add chopped parsley to blend.

4. Preheat the oven to a fan/350F of 200C/180C.

5. Put the tomato sauce to a moderate boil when you're about to prepare the beans, then switch into a shallow ovenproof bowl.

6. Crack the eggs onto the edge of the platter and gently lower them to the stew. Bake in the oven for 10-15 minutes. Cover with foil. In separate cups, eat the mixture with the eggs floating on top.

45. RAW BROWNIE BITES-NEW SIRT FOOD

Ingredients:

- 2 1/2 cups of raw walnuts

- 1/4 cup of bullets

- 2 1/2 cups date Medjool.

- 1 cup of pure cocoa

- Extract 1 teaspoon of coffee

- 1/8-1/4 tea cubicle salt.

Ingredients:

1. Place everything together in a food processor.

2. Roll in balls and put on a baker and freeze for 30 minutes or cool for 2 hours.

46. Waldorf Salad-New Sirtfood

Ingredients:

- 200 g celery, chopped

- 100 g apple, chopped

- 50 g walnuts, minced roughly

- 1 red onion, chopped roughly

- 1 chicory head, chopped

- 10 g parsley, chopped

- 1 tbsp of capers

- 10 g of lovage or celery leaves, chopped roughly

For the dressing:

- 1 tbsp of virgin-olive-oil

- 1 tbsp of balsamic vinegar

- 1 tsp of mustard Dijon

- About a lemon juice

Instructions:

1. In a medium-sized salad bowl and mix the apple, onion, celery, walnuts, caper, parsley, , and lovage. Get the dressing together by whisking the

2. Sprinkle with vinegar, sugar, lemon juice, and mustard. Blend and drink!

47. CHARGRILLED BEEF WITH A RED WINE EXTRACT, ONION RINGS, KALE AND SPICE ROASTED POTATOES-NEW SIRT FOOD

Ingredients:

- Cut 100 g potatoes in 2 cm dice

- 1 tablespoon of extra virgin olive oil

- 5 g of finely chopped parsley

- 50 g of red onion, ring-sliced

- 50 g of sliced kale

- 1 clove of garlic, finely chopped

- 120–150 g x 3.5 cm fillet steak of beef or 2 cm sirloin steak

- 40 ml of red wine

- 150ml of beef stock

- 1 tsp of mashed tomato

- Dissolved in 1 tbsp of water

- 1 tsp of corn-flour

Instructions:

1. Oven heat to 220oC / gas 7.

2. In a bowl of boiling water, bring the potatoes back to a boil, cook for 4 to 5-minutes, then drain. Put in a roasting tin with 1 teaspoon of oil and roast 35-45 minutes in the hot oven.

3. Turn the potatoes to ensure even cooking after 10 minutes. Sprinkle with chopped parsley when baked, extract from the oven and blend properly.

4. Fry the onion for 5-7 minutes in 1 teaspoon of oil until soft and nicely caramelized. Keep warm. Keep warm. Drain the kale for 2-3 minutes. In 1/2 teaspoon of oil, gently cook the garlic for 1 minute, until soft but not colored.

Attach the kale and fry until soft, for another 1–2 minutes. Keep dry. Keep moist.

5. Heat a high-heat ovenproof frying pan to smoke. Coat the meat in one half cubic meter of olive oil and fry in medium-high heat in a hot pot, according to how you like meat. In case you like your meat medium, it would be better to sew meat and transfer the pot into a 220 oC / gas seven oven and finish cooking for the prescribed times.

6. Endeavor to remove the meat from the pot and put it aside. Apply vinegar to the hot pan for any trace of beef. Bubble to halve the wine, syrupy and concentrated in flavor.

7. In the steak pan, add the pot and tomato puree and bring to boil, then add the corn-flour paste to thicken the sauce, then add it a little at a time to your desired consistency. Then, serve with the roasted potatoes, kale, onion rings, and red wine sauce in any of the juices of the steaks rested.

48. FRESH SAAG PANEER - NEW SIRT FOOD

Ingredients:

- 2 tsp of rape oil

- 200 g of Paneer. Break-in cubes

- Salt and black pepper freshly ground

- 1 red onion, freshly cut

- Fresh ginger one small thumb (3 cm), peeled and split into matches

- 1 garlic clove, skinned and finely sliced

- 1 green, desired and finely sliced chili

- Tomatoes 100 g cherry, halved

- 1/2 tsp coriander of the field

- 1/2 tsp cumin field

- 1/4 tsp turmeric on the ground

- 1/2 tsp of mild powdered chili

- 1/2 tsp of salt

- 100 g of new leaves of spinach

- A small handful (10 g), chopped parsley

- The little handful of (10 g) chopped coriander

Ingredients:

1. Over a high temperature, heat the oil over high heat in a large lidded frying pan. Add salt and pepper to the pan and toss in the pot. Fry for a few minutes, sometimes stirring before white. Take a slotted spoon from the bowl and put it aside.

2. Shrink heat and add the onion. Until incorporating ginger, garlic, and chili, fry for 5 minutes. Boil for some minutes until the cherry tomatoes are included. Place the cover on the pot and simmer for another five minutes.

3. Stir in the spices and salt. Return the bowl to the pot and mix when coated. Add the spinach and the coriander to the pot and place the lid on. Allow the spinach to wake for 1-2 minutes and then add to the dish. Serve straight away.

49. MOCHA CHOCOLATE MOUSSE-NEW SIRT FOOD

Everyone loves chocolate mousse, with wonderful light and airy feel. It's quick and simple to produce and better eaten the day it's finished.

Ingredients:

- 250 g dark chocolate (85% solid cocoa)

- medium-free, divided eggs

- 4 tbsp solid coffee black

- 4 tbsp milk of almond

- Coffee beans cream, to decorate

Instructions:

1. In a large bowl, melt the chocolate over a pot of soft water and ensure that the base of the container does not touch the water. Remove the bowl from heat and return to room temperature, the molten chocolate.

2. When the molten chocolate is room temperature, whisk one by one in the egg yolks, then add in the coffee and almond milk gently.

3. Beat the egg whites using a homemade electric mixer before steep peaks develop and then beat a few tablespoons into a chocolate mixture to loosen it. Pull the balance kindly, use a large metal spoon.

4. Transfer the mousse to each glass and smooth the surface. Top off with film and sleep, preferably overnight, for at least 2 hours. Until serving, decorate with chocolate coffee beans.

50. MUESLI BUCKWHEAT-NEW SIRT FOOD

Ingredients:

- 20 g flakes of buckwheat

- 10 g puffs of buckwheat

- 15 g chocolate flakes or chocolate desiccated

- 40 g Dates, pitted and chopped Medjool

- 15 g of walnuts, cut

- 10 g nibs of chocolate

- 100 g, hulled and chopped strawberries

- 100 g of regular Greek yogurt (or alternate vegan yogurt like tofu or cocoon)

Instructions:

Combine all of the ingredients listed above (leave strawberries and yogurt out, if not served immediately).

NOTE: To produce them in bulk or to cook them the night before, simply combine the dry ingredients in an airtight container and place them. You also have to add strawberries and milk the next day, and it's ready to go.

51.BUCKWHEAT ROLLS, DARK CHOCOLATE SYRUP, AND CRUSHED WALNUTS-NEW SIRT FOOD

You need these for the pancakes:

Ingredients:

- 350ml of meat

- 150 g of Buckwheat flour

- 1 big egg

- 1 tablespoon of extra virgin olive oil

For the sauce chocolate:

- 100 g of dark chocolate (85% solids of cocoa)

- 85 ml of milk

- 1 tbsp pair milk

- 1 tablespoon of extra virgin olive oil

To serve:

- Hulled and chopped 400 g strawberries

- 100 g walnuts, cut

Instructions:

1. Apart from the olive oil, put all the ingredients in a blender and mix until you have a smooth blend. It shouldn't be too thick or too laughable. (You can store any excess batter in an airproof container in your refrigerator for up to 5 days.

2. To produce the chocolate sauce, melt the chocolate over a saucepan of drinking water in a heatproof pot. Mix the milk once melted, whisk and then add the double cream and the olive oil.

3. You will keep the sauce warm by making the water boil on low heat in the pot before the pancakes are finished.

4. To make the pancakes heat a heavy-bottomed pan, then add the olive oil until they begin to smoke.

5. Place some of the flour in the middle of the pan and spread the extra batter around until you cover the entire surface, you may need to use a little powder to do that. You just have to cook the pancake on both sides 1 minute or so if your pot is hot enough.

6. Once you see it brown around the edges, use a paddle to loosen the pancake around its edge and turn it around. Try to reverse in one action so that it does not break down.

7. Cook for another minute and transfer to a plate on the other side.

8. In the middle, place some strawberries and roll up the pancake. Continue to create as many pancakes as possible.

9. Sprinkle a large quantity of sauce with a few chopped walnuts.

10. You can find your initial attempts too fat or fall

apart, but if you have reached your batter's rhythm, which fits well for you and has your methodology perfected, you'll become a professional. In this scenario, practice makes perfect.

52.BANANA BLUEBERRY PANCAKES WITH CHUNKY APPLE COMPOTE AND LATTE-NEW TURMERIC

Ingredients:

- ripe bananas

- 6 medium eggs

- 150 g of rolling oats

- 2 tsp flour baking

- 1/4 tea cubicle oil.

- 25 g of blueberries

For the Apple Chunky Compote

- 2 of apples

- 5 of (pitted) dates

- 1 tbsp lemon juice

- ¼ tbsp of cinnamon powder

- Sprinkle with salt

For the Golden Latte Turmeric

- 3 cups of powdered powder

- 1 turmeric tablespoon powder

- 1 teaspoon cinnamon powder

- 1 tablespoon of organic sweetheart

- Black pepper (increased absorption)

- The small new, peeled root of ginger

- Cayenne pepper pick (optional)

Instructions:

For the Banana Blueberry Pancakes

1. Pop the rolled oats into a high-speed mixer and pulse 1 minute or until the flour of the oat are formed.

Tip: Ensure your blender is very dry, or everything is going to become soggy before doing this!

1. Add to the blender now bananas, eggs, baking

powder, and salt and pulse for 2 minutes until it forms a smooth batter.

2. Transfer the blueberries in a large bowl and fold. Enable 10 minutes to rest while the baking powder clicks on.

3. To make the pancakes, apply a dollar of butter (this makes them tasty and crispy!) on medium-high heat to your frying pan. Add a few spoons to the mixture of the blueberry pancakes and fry until the bottom is very golden. Throw the pancake on the other side to fry.

With the Apple Chunky Compote

1. Roughly chop your apples

2. Pop all along with two teaspoons of water and a sprinkle of salt in a food processor. Pulse your chunky compote apple to shape.

For the Golden Latte Turmeric

1. Mix all the ingredients in a high-speed blender until smooth.

2. Put in a tiny saucepan and cook over medium heat for 4 minutes until hot but not boiling. Enjoy!

53. BLUEBERRY SMOOTHIE - NEW SIRT FOOD

This smoothie Yogurt has a rich, creamy flavor.

Ingredients:

- 1 big ripe banana

- 100 g of blueberries

- 100 g of blackberries

- 2 tbsp of yogurt

- 200ml of dairy milk

Instructions:

Mix together all ingredients until smooth.

54. LEMON YOGURT SAUCE-WITH SAVORY TURMERIC PANCAKES-NEW SIRT FOOD

Ingredients:

For the sauce with Yogurt:

- 1 cup of Greek straight yogurt

- 1 hairy garlic clove

- 1-2 tbsp of Lemon juice to taste

- 1/4 tea cubicle ground turmeric

- 10 fresh, thinned mint leaves

- 2 citrus zest teaspoons (1 lemon)

For Pancakes:

- 2 teaspoons of turmeric (grounded)

- 1 1/2 ground cumin teaspoons

- 1 tsp of salt

- 1 tablespoon coriander (grounded)

- 1/2 tea cubicle garlic powder.

- Fresh ground black pepper 1/2 teaspoon

- 1 head of broccoli, cut into blooms

- 3 big eggs, slightly beaten

- 2 tablespoons unflavored almond milk

- 1 cup of amber meal.

- 4 tea cubes of cocoa butter

Instructions:

1. Make the sauce for yogurt. In a cup, mix milk, ginger, citrus oil, turmeric, mint, and zest. Flavor and season, if needed, with more lemon juice. Place aside or cool until ready to serve.

2 . Make your pancakes. 2. Combine turmeric, cumin, cinnamon, coriander, garlic, and pepper in a tiny pot.

3. Place broccoli in the food processor and pulse it into small pieces until the blooms are broken up. Transfer broccoli to a big bowl, add eggs, almond milk, and meal of almond. Remove the spice mixture and mix well.

4. Heat 1-teaspoon of coconut oil in a medium-low heat non-stick pan. Put 1/4 cup of batter into the pot. Cook the bacon before tiny bubbles emerge on the top and golden brown on the bottom for 2 to 3 minutes. Make/cook the pancake for another 2 to 3 minutes. To stay warm, through the cooked pancakes in a 200°F oven with an oven-safe.

The remaining three pancakes continue to be made with the remaining oil and syrup. 5.

178

55. CHILI CON CARNE-NEW SIRT FOOD

Ingredients:

- 1 red onion, thinly sliced.

- 3 cloves of garlic, finely chopped

- 2 chilies with bird's eye, finely chopped

- 1 tbsp of extra virgin olive oil

- 1 tbsp cumin ground

- 1 tbsp turmeric powder

- 400 g of lean beef (5% fat)

- 50 ml of red wine

- 1 red pepper, cored, removed seeds, and cut into pieces of bite.

- Tomatoes sliced 2 x 400 g

- 1 tbsp of pureed tomato.

- 1 tbsp powder of cocoa

- 150 g of kidney beans tinned

- 300ml of stock of beef

- 5 g of chopped coriander

- 5 g of parsley

- 160 g of buckwheat

Ingredients:

1. In a saucepan, spray the onion, garlic, and chili in the oil 2-3 minutes, then add the spices and simmer one minute in medium heat.

2. Attach the tall, brown beef to medium-high heat. Put the red wine and allow it to bubble to halve it.

3. Stir in the red pepper, onions, puree, coffee, kidney, and stock and simmer for 1 hour.

4. However, you might need to add some water to get a thick, sticky consistency.

5. Drop the chopped herbs just before eating.

6. In the meantime, cook the buckwheat and serve with the chili according to the packet instructions.

56 CHICKPEA, QUINOA AND TURMERIC CURRY-NEW SIRT FOOD RECIPES

Ingredients:

- Halved 500 g of new potatoes

- 3 cloves of garlic, crushed

- 3 ground turmeric teaspoons

- 1 tablespoon coriander (ground)

- 1 teaspoon of liquid chili flakes

- 1 ground ginger teaspoon

- 400 g cocoa milk can

- 1 tbsp of puree tomato.

- 400 g can of tomatoes diced

- Pepper and salt

- 180 g of quinoa

- 400 g of Chickpeas rinsed and drained

- 150 g of spinach

-

Instructions:

1. Place-the-potatoes in a pot of cold water and bring them to a boil. Cook for around 25 minutes so you can comfortably run a knife through them. Drain them well. Drain them well.

2. In a large pot, add garlic, turmeric, coriander, chili, ginger, coconut milk, tomato puree, and tomatoes. Bring the salt and pepper to the boil, then add the quinoa with a mug of boiled water (300 ml).

3. Reduce the heat to cool, place the cover on, and cool. Make sure you stir every 5 minutes for the next 30 minutes to make sure nothing stays down. (It's a quite long kitchen time, but how long it takes for the quinoa to cook in all these ingredients instead of just water.) When only 5 minutes remain, attach the spinach and blend until wilted. It is ready when the quinoa is cooked and smooth, not crunchy.

4. If you like a little fire, apply a red slice of chili

to the curry and the other spices simultaneously.

CONCLUSION

Sirtfood Diet is the latest approach to a quick weight loss without an extreme diet by triggering the same 'skinny gene' mechanisms, usually just through exercise and fasting. Some foods contain chemical substances known as polyphenols that stress our cells mildly, enabling genes to imitate the effects of exercise and fasting. The Sirtuin pathways, which affect metabolism, age, and mood, are guided by the food rich in polyphenols, like broccoli, dark chocolate, and red wine. However, a diet sufficient in these Sirtfoods starts to lose weight without sacrificing muscle while maintaining excellent health.

Combine healthy Sirtfoods with efficient and sustained weight loss, great energy, and bright health to your diet. Switch on the fat-burning strength, overburden weight loss, and help stave off disease with this easy-to-follow diet that nutritional, medical experts have established who have demonstrated the impact of Sirtfoods. Dark chocolate, coffee, and kale – they are all menus that enable Sirtuin and switch to what is known as 'skinny gene' in the body. Sirtfood Diet presents you with a fast and safe way to eat for weight reduction, delicious easy-to-make recipes, and a long-term performance management program. The Sirtfood Diet is an inclusion diet without exclusion, and Sirtfood is widely available and affordable. However, this is a diet that encourages you to get a better version of yourself.

www.ingramcontent.com/pod-product-compliance
Lightning Source LLC
Chambersburg PA
CBHW072222150726

48002CB00005B/1930